Renal Cell Carcinoma - Recent Advances, New Perspectives and Applications

Edited by Jindong Chen

Published in London, United Kingdom

Renal Cell Carcinoma - Recent Advances, New Perspectives and Applications
http://dx.doi.org/10.5772/intechopen.102246
Edited by Jindong Chen

Contributors
Mary Taub, Vaidehi Alpesh Patel, Shuji Isotani, Helge Waldum, Patricia Mjønes, Yichun Zheng, Chengcheng Xing, Dekai Liu, Jiaqi Du, Gangfu Zheng, Nengfeng Yu, Dingya Zhou, Honghui Cheng, Kefan Yang, Qifeng Zhong, Congcong Xu, Jindong Chen

First published in London, United Kingdom, 2023 by IntechOpen
IntechOpen is the global imprint of INTECHOPEN LIMITED, registered in England and Wales, registration number: 11086078, 5 Princes Gate Court, London, SW7 2QJ, United Kingdom

British Library Cataloguing-in-Publication Data
A catalogue record for this book is available from the British Library

Additional hard and PDF copies can be obtained from orders@intechopen.com

Renal Cell Carcinoma - Recent Advances, New Perspectives and Applications
Edited by Jindong Chen
p. cm.
Print ISBN 978-1-83969-469-1
Online ISBN 978-1-83969-470-7
eBook (PDF) ISBN 978-1-83969-471-4

Meet the editor

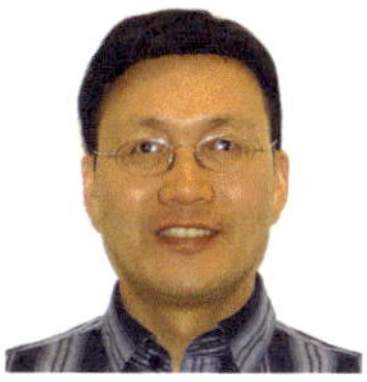

Jindong Chen earned his Ph.D. from the Karolinska Institute, Sweden. He is an active member of the American Association for Cancer Research (AACR) and the chief technology officer at Exploring Health, LLC. He is also a professor at Zunyi Medical University, China, and a former research associate professor and kidney laboratory co-director at the University of Rochester Medical Center, USA. When serving as a research scientist at Van Andel Research Institute, USA, and a senior scientist at the National Cancer Center Singapore and Duke-NUS University Medical School, USA, Dr. Chen position-cloned two cancer-related genes, *NORE1* and *LSAMP*, and participated in the identification of *HRPT2* and *FLCN*. He subsequently developed several *FLCN* and *HRPT2* knockout mouse models. For those achievements, he was awarded at the 94th and 100th AACR annual meetings. Currently, Dr. Chen is working on the development of anti-metastasis drugs.

Contents

Preface

Kidney cancer is the sixth most common malignant disease in men and the tenth most common in women. It accounts for 5% of male and 3% of female malignancies. With the development and improvement of new techniques, updated knowledge and information are essential for the management of renal cell carcinoma (RCC).

In the past decade, the use of improved diagnostic methods such as ultrasound, contrast-enhanced ultrasound (CEUS), computed tomography (CT) scan, magnetic resonance imaging (MRI), and positron emission tomography (PET)/CT scan has significantly increased the detection rate of RCC. Additionally, robotic platforms with the integration of imaging approaches have been adopted in RCC surgery, which has transformed the paradigm in the surgical treatment of RCC and will continue to change it in the future. With the use of robot-assisted partial nephrectomy in RCC surgery, urologists can maximize functional and oncologic outcomes in nephron preservation and complication-free recovery. For advanced or metastatic RCC, the progress in targeted therapy, immunotherapy, and combination therapy has been improving patient survival outcomes. For these reasons, the mortality of RCC has been decreasing although its incidence is increasing.

With international experts sharing their experience, knowledge, and review, this book provides updated information on the epidemiology, genetics, diagnosis, screening, and advances in treatment and management of RCC to treating physicians as well as their patients. The book is also a useful resource for researchers in the field.

I would like to give my sincere thanks to all the contributing authors as well as the team at IntechOpen, especially Author Service Manager Ms. Martina Scerbe and Publishing Process Manager Ms. Paula Gavran. Without their support, dedication, and effort, this book would not have been possible.

Jindong Chen
Chief Technology Officer,
Exploring Health, LLC
Guangzhou, China

Section 1

Diagnosis of Renal Cell Carcinoma

Chapter 1

Perspective Chapter: An Update on Renal Cell Carcinoma

Jindong Chen

Abstract

Incidence and mortality of renal cell carcinoma (RCC) significantly vary worldwide. While RCC incidence has been increasing, its mortality rate has been decreasing. Smoking, obesity, hypertension, chronic kidney disease (CKD), ethnicity, location, and other environmental factors are reported to be associated with RCC. With the use of the improved diagnostic methods, including ultrasound, contrast-enhanced ultrasound (CEUS), computed tomography (CT) scan, magnetic resonance imaging (MRI), and positron emission tomography (PET)/CT scan, the detection rate of RCC has significantly increased over the past decade. We have witnessed innovation in surgical techniques and robotic platforms with integration of imaging approaches, and urologists are now able to maximize functional and oncologic outcomes in nephron preservation and complication-free recovery. Thus, the paradigm in the surgical treatment of RCC has transformed and will continue to change in the future. In addition, targeted therapy, immunotherapy, and combination therapy are adopted to treat patients with advanced RCC. In recent years, the combination of immune checkpoint inhibition and antiangiogenic therapy is a very attractive combined therapeutic strategy for advanced/metastatic RCCs. Biomarkers, including epigenetic markers for RCC, have been increasing, which will be helpful to discover new therapeutic targets and related inhibitors for the treatment of advanced RCC.

Keywords: kidney cancer, renal cell carcinoma, RCC, genetics, targeted therapy, immunotherapy, combination therapy

1. Introduction

Kidney cancer has been known to have distinct histological types with different genetic profiles. The most common type is renal cell carcinoma (RCC), representing more than 90% of all kidney cancers [1]. RCC is consisted of a few subtypes. The most common subtype is clear cell renal cell carcinoma (ccRCC), followed by papillary RCC (pRCC, type I and type II), chromophobe RCC (cRCC), collecting duct carcinoma (CDC), etc. Kidney cancer is the sixth most common malignant disease in men and tenth in women. It accounts for 5% of male and 3% female malignancies [2, 3]. The RCC incidence is constantly rising as well. In urology, kidney cancer is the third most common malignant disease. While kidney cancer occurs mostly in North American and European, the incidence of renal cancer is relatively lower in Asian [4]. Based on the global cancer statistics in 2020 [5, 6], there were an estimated 431,300 people diagnosed with kidney cancer and approximately 179,400 deaths worldwide in 2020. It was recently estimated that there were 81,800 new kidney cancer cases and 14,890 deaths in the United States in 2023 [7]. Diagnosis of RCC at early stages is crucial in treating patients and improving survival rates. With the application of improved diagnostic techniques such as cross-section abdominal imaging [8], the detection rate of RCC has increased in recent years [9]. Choosing the best therapeutic strategy is essential for improving the outcome of patients with RCC.

2. Epidemiology of RCC

RCC is the most lethal urogenital cancer, accounting for 2–3% of all cancers. The incidence of RCC is continuously rising worldwide, and it is higher in developed countries compared to developing countries, and higher in men than women (male to female ratio is 1.5:1). The mortality rate of RCC is 30–40% and is higher in men compared to women [3]. The majority of RCC patients are aged over 60 years. Since the advance in diagnostic methods and public consciousness of the importance of periodic health screening, the number of RCC patients diagnosed in the early stages keeps increasing. Thus, the incidence of RCC has been rising as well in the past three decades [9]. Even though, the mortality rate of RCC has been constantly decreasing, especially in developed countries, due to early therapy and progress of the therapeutic strategies [10]. However, despite the improvement in disease control and increased survival rate, metastases are often observed in many RCC patients [11]. As reported, 30–50% of patients with local RCC progress to metastasis. In addition, metastasis was observed in 20–30% of the RCC patients at the early stage of diagnosis, and nearly 40% of the patients with localized RCC tumors presented distant metastases even after surgery. The most common distant metastatic sites are the lungs, bones (vertebrae, proximal part of the femur, pelvic bones), lymphatic nodes brain, liver, the opposite kidney, and suprarenal glands [12]. The patients with RCC metastases suffer from pain, nerve compression, hypercalcemia, and pathological fractures. The occurrence of metastases often worsens the patients' prognosis [13]. The median survival for patients with RCC metastases is approximately 8 months and the mortality rate is 50% during the first year, and 10% for 5 years survival [10, 13, 14].

3. Risk factors associated with RCC

While age and gender are strongly associated with increased RCC incidence, hypertension, smoking, obesity, ethnicity, location, and history of using tobacco products increase the risk of RCC as well [3]. It was reported that smoking could increase the risk by about 54% in men and 22% in women. Smoking time and the daily number of cigarettes are directly associated with kidney cancer incidence for both men and women. In addition, some minor risk factors that may be related to RCC include acquired renal cystic disease, chronic kidney disease (CKD), end-stage renal disease (ESRD), exposure to cadmium and trichloroethylene, consumption of red and processed meat, chronic use of palliatives, type-2 diabetes, vitamin D level, viral hepatitis, increased triglycerides, decreased physical activity, and genetic syndromes [15]. Patients with renal insufficiency and in the terminal stage of the disease are four times more likely to develop kidney cancer. Measures of preventing RCC include smoking cessation, and reducing of the body mass index (BMI), etc.

4. Pathophysiology of RCC

Since RCC is a heterogeneous cancer that may stem from different type of renal cells, histological subtyping of RCC may exert a crucial impact on the choice of therapeutic strategies and prognosis. Based on the histological features, RCC is divided into 16 subtypes, including clear cell RCC, pRCC (type I and II), cRCC, collecting duct RCC, multilocular cystic RCC, medullary carcinoma, mucinous tubular, spindle cell carcinoma, neuroblastoma-associated RCC, Xp11.2 translocations—TFE3 carcinoma, hereditary cancer syndromes, and unclassified lesion [16]. Of them, clear cell RCC is the most common subtype of RCC and accounts for 75–85%. The second most common one is pRCC that constitutes 10–15%. cRCC ranked third and represents 3–5% of kidney cancers. Both clear cell carcinoma and pRCC are thought to stem from the proximal tubule, while chromophore RCC originates from the distal connecting tubules (DCT) and collecting duct system, especially the intercalated cells [17]. While most clear cell RCCs are sporadic, approximately 5% of the clear cell RCC is hereditary, and usually related to hereditary syndromes such as Von Hippel–Lindau disease (VHL) and tuberous sclerosis (TS). Clear cell RCC tends to metastasize to the lymph nodes, the lungs, the liver, and bones. Clear cell RCC has poorer prognosis compared to pRCC and cRCC. On the basis of histological and genetic differences, pRCC is further divided into two subtypes: type I and type II. The type I pRCC cannot be distinguished from type II through routine imaging techniques. Papillary type I can be detected at an early stage, and thus has a better prognosis compared to type II. cRCC is commonly observed in patients aged more than 60, and less aggressive compared to clear cell RCC. Therefore, cRCC has the best prognosis among all RCCs [4].

5. Genetics of RCC

The first categorization of kidney cancer based on molecular genetics was conducted by Heidelberg in 1997, and it was adopted in the WHO tumor classification of 2004, 2012 Vancouver ISUP [18], and the latest RCC classification of the WHO (2016) [16]. RCC has various genetic alterations, including gene mutations, epigenetic modifications, and chromosomal aberrations. While genetic alterations can cause both sporadic and hereditary types, patients with familial history (hereditary) represent only 3% of all kidney cancer cases. An increased number of RCC-related genes were identified in the past decades. Considering its high genetic heterogeneity, RCC can be caused by mutations in many genes and chromosomal abnormalities. Each subtype of RCC has its corresponding affected genes [19]. Clear cell RCC-related genes include *VHL*, *PBRM1, BAP1, STED2, JARID1c*, *FLCN*, and c-MYC. *VHL* mutations account for approximately 60% of clear cell RCC [20]. In addition, exome-sequencing has revealed that *PBRM1, SETD2, BAP1, and JARID1c* are associated with RCC as well (*PBRM1,* 40%, *SETD2,* 12%, *BAP1,*10%, and *KDM5C,*5%) [21]. Combinational mutations of the above genes were also detected in many clear cell RCCs. With the advent of new genetic tools, more RCC-related genes/biomarkers might be uncovered.

pRCC is divided into two types: Type I and Type II. Although pRCC type I and type II are morphologically similar, they are cytologically different. Compare to pRCC II, pRCC type I has a low-grade tendency and better prognosis [22]. pRCC I is often caused by overexpression of the *MET* gene on chromosome 7q31, while pRCC II is less correlated to MET overexpression but associated with alterations in *FH*, *CDKN2A*, *SETD2*, *BAP1*, *PBRM1*, *FLCN*, *NRF2-ARE*, *TERT*, *TFE3*, and increased expression of *NF2* [23, 24]. cRCC is a relatively rare type of RCC that originates from the distal convoluted tubule. cRCC is associated with mutations in *PTEN*, *TP53*, *mTOR*, *c-kit*, *FAAH2*, *PDHB*, *PDXD1*, *ZNF765*, *PRKAG2*, *ARID1A*, and *ABHD3*. Of them, *PTEN* mutation is the most common event in cRCC [25]. In addition, mutations in *FLCN* appear to cause all types of RCC in *Flcn* knockout mouse models [26, 27].

Chromosomal aberration is also a common feature in RCC [28]. In clear cell RCC, the loss of the short arm of chromosome 3 is the most frequently occurred event, which is related to the loss of the *VHL* gene located on 3p [28, 29]. Other chromosomal aberrations include loss of chromosome Y, gaining 5q31, 8q, 4p, 14q, 9p, and trisomy of chromosome 7. Patients with gaining of 4p, 9p, and 14q have poor prognosis while gaining 5q31 is connected with prolonged survival in high-grade clear cell RCC. Deletion of the Y chromosome usually leads to clear cell RCC with distant metastasis. In addition, gaining chromosome 8q can cause metastasis of clear cell RCC, which may be associated with overexpression of C-MYC. For chromosomal abnormity, pRCC type I is also different from papillary type II. Trisomy of chromosomes (e.g., 3q, 7, 8, 12, 16, 17, 20) commonly appears in type I pRCC. In addition, loss of chromosome Y is an important feature of papillary type II in men. In contrast, gaining a chromosome 8q and losing 1p and 9p are frequently observed in RCC papillary type II. cRCC is also associated with chromosome aberrations, including loss of chromosomes 1, 2, 6, 10, 13, 17, and 21 [20]. Losing copies of chromosomes 1, 2, 6, 10, 13, and 17 are more commonly observed in the classical type of cRCC than the eosinophilic type [30]. In addition, gaining chromosome copies (e.g., 4, 7, 11, 12, 14q, and 18q) is related to cRCC as well [31].

6. Clinical diagnosis of RCC

Since small RCC masses are usually asymptomatic, the majority of RCCs are accidentally detected by routine imaging for various medical screening purposes [32]. Patients diagnosed with RCC based on the symptoms account for only 30%, and approximately 20–30% of the patients present metastasis at the time of diagnosis. Flank pain, hematuria, and abdominal mass are usually considered as the classic symptoms for RCC diagnosis, but these symptoms are observed in only 4–17% of the cases. Other symptoms for diagnosis include fever, abdominal pain, anemia-induced fatigue, weight loss, bone pain, and cough caused by metastasis of cancer cells or lower limb edema, peripheral lymphadenopathy (LAP), and varicocele caused by inferior vena cava (IVC) or renal thrombosis [33]. Once signs and symptoms appear, further laboratory investigation should be performed. The laboratory investigation includes renal function tests, complete blood cell count (CBC), liver function tests, urinary analysis, thyroid function tests, and examination of the level of calcium, lactate dehydrogenase, and alkaline phosphatase.

Various preclinical imaging modalities are valuable tools for detecting renal masses. These imaging modalities include ultrasound, CEUS, computed tomography (CT) scan, magnetic resonance imaging (MRI), positron emission tomography

(PET)/CT, etc. Many renal masses and benign cystic kidney lesions can be easily detected with ultrasound [34]. In addition, as an inexpensive and accurate imaging approach, contrast-enhanced ultrasound (CEUS) has been adopted to evaluate indeterminate renal lesions, though it may not effectively discriminate between malignant and benign renal masses. For more accurately identifying malignant masses, CT scan or MRI is required [35]. In some cases, both CT and MRI should be performed by contrast because contrast absorption is a key factor in determining malignant masses [36]. For small lesions (1–2 cm) and in cases of renal insufficiency, pregnant women, and patients allergic to contrast material, MRI should be conducted [37]. The primary purpose of imaging is to inspect the characteristics of the affected mass, identify possible abdominal metastases, mass expansion, and venous involvement for staging. PET scan, is not a standard scan strategy, is very helpful in the diagnosis and follow-up of RCC. Thus, routine use of PET/CT is also recommended [38]. Other imaging approaches, including advanced MRI techniques or the combination use of iodine PET and CT, may be performed to determine renal masses [39]. In addition, biopsy and histopathology are required to carry out in suspected masses before further treatment.

7. Treatment and management of RCC

To date, surgery is still an essential treatment for RCC, and RE nephrectomy has been regarded as the standard of care for the management of renal tumors. For small renal lesions and surgery-induced chronic kidney disorders, active surveillance of nephron surgery and minimally invasive approaches have been adopted to limit the invasion and loss of kidney function in clinical [40]. RCC patients with severe comorbidities, elderly patients with small tumors ≤4 cm, or patients with a short life expectancy are recommended for active surveillance [41]. In some cases, active surveillance is also suggested to monitor the rate of the large tumor's growth. In addition, imaging can be performed for active surveillance in the first half year, and then, every 6 months at 2–3 years, and later, annually [42]. In addition, for treating small randomly detected tumors, minimally invasive procedures should be used. Cryotherapy (CRYO) and radiofrequency ablations (RFA) were suggested for patients with only one kidney or for those unable to undergo major surgery.

7.1 Nephron preservation surgery

While radical nephrectomy is the removal of the entire kidney and is suitable for patients with larger renal tumors (T2, >7 cm), nephron-sparing partial nephrectomy only removes the small localized renal tumor (T1, <7 cm) and preserves the parenchyma. Thus, in most cases including locally advanced and metastatic diseases, nephron-sparing partial nephrectomy is recommended except for those that technically impossible to be removed due to their unfavorable location.

The advent and improvement of robot-assisted surgical approaches and robotic platforms have helped to close the technical gap and allow for greater adoption of the laparoscopic approach and nephron-sparing surgery, leading to a revolution for surgical management of RCC in recent decades [43, 44]. As the use of robotic platforms combined with imaging techniques in surgery, larger, higher stage, and more complex renal lesions can now be treated in a minimally invasive fashion, which leads to decreased morbidity, shortened patients' hospitalization, and less side effects [45, 46].

Robot-assisted surgery has continued to evolve and has been playing an ever-expanding role in the treatment of RCC worldwide [45]. Laparoscopic partial nephrectomy and robot-assisted partial nephrectomy are becoming the standard treatment for patients eligible for nephron-sparing surgery. While the nephron-sparing surgery has been endorsed as the gold standard treatment of T1a tumors ≤4 cm in size and T1b lesions in the United States and Europe when technically possible with experienced surgeons [41, 47], robot-assisted partial nephrectomy has been adopted for treatment of cT2 RCC [48]. While new robotic platforms such as single-port (SP) robotic surgical system and multiport robotic surgical systems are currently under development, the popular da Vinci platform has significantly expanded the laparoscopic paradigm spectrum in the surgical treatment of RCC [49–51].

7.2 Cytokine treatment of metastatic disease

Before targeted therapy, patients with metastatic clear cell RCC were previously treated with immunosuppressive agents such as INFα and IL2, namely systemic therapy. In 1990s, systemic therapy with a high-dose IL2 turned into a commonly used modality for various cancer patients with metastasis. However, complete response was only observed in <10% of patients treated with a longer high dose of IL-2. It simultaneously caused severe toxic effects. Thus, high-dose IL2 treatment is not recommended for patients with metastatic RCC unless the patients are young and in very good conditions with low tumor volume [52].

Aldesleukin and INFα (along with Bevacizumab) are the only safe modulating drugs that are approved in selected metastatic RCC. INFα is adopted to treat RCC patients in various formulas with a response rate of 10–15% and a response time of 4 months. Patients who benefit from INF treatment were then subjected to nephrectomy. Although INFα treatment shows some efficacy in the treatment of patients with metastatic RCC, it is not suggested for treating RCC patients as a single drug.

7.3 Targeted therapy and immunotherapy of metastatic RCC

In the past decades, the most significant advance in the therapeutic strategy of metastatic RCC has been the development of treatments that specifically target the RCC-related biological pathways and related biomarkers [53, 54]. In the 1990s, cytokines, such as IFNα and IL-2, were used to treat metastatic clear cell RCC (**Figure 1**). In the 2000s, targeted therapies that target the VEGF/PDGFR/mTOR pathways replaced the cytokine therapies. In the targeted therapies, tyrosine kinase inhibitors (TKIs) are effective agents in the treatment of metastatic RCC, which was used as the first line and the second line treatment options. To date, five TKIs (e.g., cabozantinib, axitinib, pazopanib, sorafenib, and sunitinib) have been approved internationally for the targeted therapy of metastatic RCC (**Figure 1**). Cabozantinib targets the tyrosine-protein kinase receptor UFO and the MET receptor tyrosine kinase. Pazopanib targets the VEGFR, while axitinib inhibits VEGFR with improved specificity, sorafenib an multi-kinase inhibitor, inhibits RAF-1, B-RAF, VEGFR-2, VEGFR-3, PDGF-β, KIT, and FLT-3. Sunitinib targets VEGFR2(Flk-1) and PDGFR-β. Whereas, lenvatinib suppresses VEGFRs and fibroblast growth factor receptors [55, 56]. In addition, temsirolimus and everolimus, two mTOR inhibitors, have been approved for the treatment of advanced RCC as well. Bevacizumab, an anti-VEGF monoclonal antibody, is approved for the treatment of advanced RCC when it is used in combination with INF. In 2015, nivolumab, an anti-PD-1 immune checkpoint

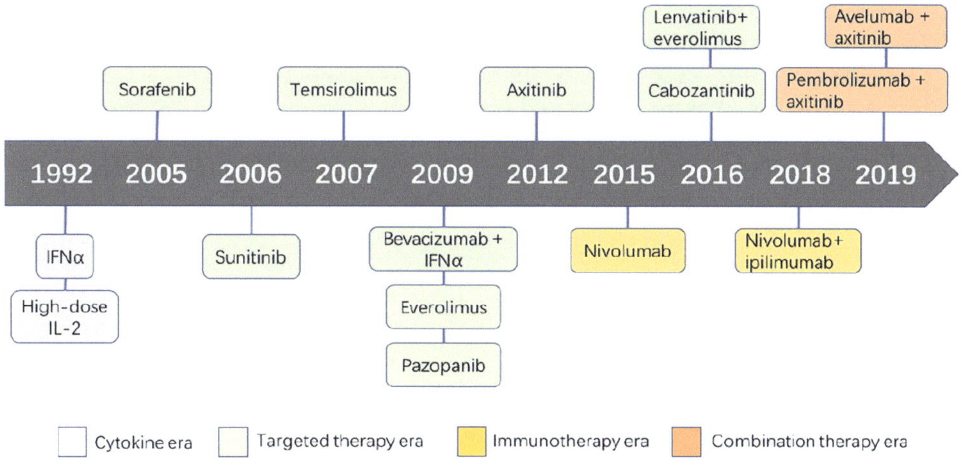

Figure 1.
Development of approved anti-RCC agents.

inhibitor that prevents signaling through programmed cell death 1, has been approved for the first immunotherapy agent of metastatic RCC [57]. Later, ipilimumab, an anti-CTLA-4 monoclonal antibody, in combination with nivolumab was approved for the first-line treatment of advanced RCC [20, 58]. Recently, increasing attention has been paid to the combination therapy. The latest combination therapy strategies such as axitinib–avelumab (target VEGF and immune checkpoints) [59, 60], axitinib–pembrolizumab (target VEGFR) in combination with PD-L1 and PD-1, respectively, have been used to treat metastatic RCC. To date, immune checkpoint inhibition plus antiangiogenic therapy constitutes a very promising combined therapeutic strategy for advanced/metastatic RCCs.

In addition, some epigenetic markers have been proposed as promising epigenetic RCC markers based on DNA methylation, ncRNA expression, and histone modification [61–63]. Many epigenetic markers and epigenetic modifiers are likely candidates for clinical use, but further validation is needed [63, 64]. The development of epigenetic therapies, either alone or in combination with antiangiogenic agents and/or immune-checkpoint inhibitors, is a hopeful therapeutic strategy for RCC.

8. Conclusion

RCC accounts for 4%of all malignant tumors. In urology, RCC is the third most common malignant tumor. Risk factors include positive family history, smoking, obesity, high blood pressure, etc. Although most cases of RCC are diagnosed accidentally, the improvement in diagnostic approaches has increased the detection rate over the past decades. Many RCC-related genes and predictive biomarkers are being identified and may further improve the diagnosis of RCC. In addition, choosing the best therapeutic strategy is critical to improve the outcome of RCC. The tumor size, the stage of the disorder, and the surgeon's experience are the determinant impact factors in the choice of the optimal treatment approach. While the open surgery is still reserved for locally advanced diseases, it is gradually displaced by robotic-assisted partial nephrectomy. Although the optimal first-line treatment, including targeted therapy, immunotherapy, or combined therapy for metastatic RCC may differ by clinical risk group and efficacy endpoint, the first-line treatment landscape for metastatic RCC is rapidly evolving. Thus, knowledge of the latest advances in the diagnosis and management of RCC could assist the related researchers, physicians, and nephrologists, to better diagnose and treat RCC.

Author details

Jindong Chen
Exploring Health, LLC., Guangzhou, Guangdong, China

*Address all correspondence to: jindong_chen@hotmail.com

References

[1] Hsieh JJ, Purdue MP, Signoretti S, Swanton C, Albiges L, Schmidinger M, et al. Renal cell carcinoma. Nature Reviews. Disease Primers. 2017;**3**:17009

[2] Miller KD, Goding Sauer A, Ortiz AP, Fedewa SA, Pinheiro PS, Tortolero-Luna G, et al. Cancer statistics for hispanics/latinos, 2018. CA: A Cancer Journal for Clinicians. 2018;**68**(6):425-445

[3] Bahadoram S, Davoodi M, Hassanzadeh S, Bahadoram M, Barahman M, Mafakher L. Renal cell carcinoma: An overview of the epidemiology, diagnosis, and treatment. Giornale Italiano di Nefrologia. 2022;**39**(3)

[4] Capitanio U, Bensalah K, Bex A, Boorjian SA, Bray F, Coleman J, et al. Epidemiology of renal cell carcinoma. European Urology. 2019;**75**(1):74-84

[5] Siegel RL, Miller KD, Jemal A. Cancer statistics, 2020. CA: A Cancer Journal for Clinicians. 2020;**70**(1):7-30

[6] Sung H, Ferlay J, Siegel RL, Laversanne M, Soerjomataram I, Jemal A, et al. Global Cancer Statistics 2020: GLOBOCAN estimates of incidence and mortality worldwide for 36 cancers in 185 countries. CA: A Cancer Journal for Clinicians. 2021;**71**(3):209-249

[7] Siegel RL, Miller KD, Wagle NS, Jemal A. Cancer statistics, 2023. CA: A Cancer Journal for Clinicians. 2023;**73**(1):17-48

[8] Kane CJ, Mallin K, Ritchey J, Cooperberg MR, Carroll PR. Renal cell cancer stage migration: analysis of the National Cancer Data Base. Cancer. 2008;**113**(1):78-83

[9] Ljungberg B, Campbell SC, Choi HY, Jacqmin D, Lee JE, Weikert S, et al. The epidemiology of renal cell carcinoma. European Urology. 2011;**60**(4):615-621

[10] Medina-Rico M, Ramos HL, Lobo M, Romo J, Prada JG. Epidemiology of renal cancer in developing countries: review of the literature. Canadian Urological Association Journal. 2018;**12**(3):E154-E162

[11] Vasudev NS, Wilson M, Stewart GD, Adeyoju A, Cartledge J, Kimuli M, et al. Challenges of early renal cancer detection: symptom patterns and incidental diagnosis rate in a multicentre prospective UK cohort of patients presenting with suspected renal cancer. BMJ Open. 2020;**10**(5):e035938

[12] Ather MH, Masood N, Siddiqui T. Current management of advanced and metastatic renal cell carcinoma. Urology Journal. 2010;7(1):1-9

[13] Umer M, Mohib Y, Atif M, Nazim M. Skeletal metastasis in renal cell carcinoma: a review. Ann Med Surg (Lond). 2018;**27**:9-16

[14] Dovalova D, Rybar L, El Falougy H, Kubikova E, Mifkovic A. Renal cell carcinoma - summarizing overview, biomarkers, metastases and new perspectives. Bratislavské Lekárske Listy. 2022;**123**(10):697-704

[15] Choueiri TK, Je Y, Cho E. Analgesic use and the risk of kidney cancer: a meta-analysis of epidemiologic studies. International Journal of Cancer. 2014;**134**(2):384-396

[16] Moch H, Cubilla AL, Humphrey PA, Reuter VE, Ulbright TM. The 2016 WHO classification of tumours of the urinary

system and male genital organs - Part A: renal, penile, and testicular tumours. European Urology. 2016;**70**(1):93-105

[17] Warren AY, Harrison D. WHO/ISUP classification, grading and pathological staging of renal cell carcinoma: standards and controversies. World Journal of Urology. 2018;**36**(12):1913-1926

[18] Delahunt B, Srigley JR, Montironi R, Egevad L. Advances in renal neoplasia: recommendations from the 2012 International Society of Urological Pathology Consensus Conference. Urology. 2014;**83**(5):969-974

[19] Cairns P. Renal cell carcinoma. Cancer Biomarkers. 2010;**9**(1-6):461-473

[20] Maher ER. Hereditary renal cell carcinoma syndromes: diagnosis, surveillance and management. World Journal of Urology. 2018;**36**(12):1891-1898

[21] Varela I, Tarpey P, Raine K, Huang D, Ong CK, Stephens P, et al. Exome sequencing identifies frequent mutation of the SWI/SNF complex gene PBRM1 in renal carcinoma. Nature. 2011;**469**(7331):539-542

[22] Klatte T, Rao PN, de Martino M, LaRochelle J, Shuch B, Zomorodian N, et al. Cytogenetic profile predicts prognosis of patients with clear cell renal cell carcinoma. Journal of Clinical Oncology. 2009;**27**(5):746-753

[23] Tovar EA, Graveel CR. MET in human cancer: germline and somatic mutations. Annals of Translational Medicine. 2017;**5**(10):205

[24] Furge KA, Chen J, Koeman J, Swiatek P, Dykema K, Lucin K, et al. Detection of DNA copy number changes and oncogenic signaling abnormalities from gene expression data reveals MYC activation in high-grade papillary renal cell carcinoma. Cancer Research. 2007;**67**(7):3171-3176

[25] Durinck S, Stawiski EW, Pavia-Jimenez A, Modrusan Z, Kapur P, Jaiswal BS, et al. Spectrum of diverse genomic alterations define non-clear cell renal carcinoma subtypes. Nature Genetics. 2015;**47**(1):13-21

[26] Chen J, Futami K, Petillo D, Peng J, Wang P, Knol J, et al. Deficiency of FLCN in mouse kidney led to development of polycystic kidneys and renal neoplasia. PLoS One. 2008;**3**(10):e3581

[27] Chen J, Huang D, Rubera I, Futami K, Wang P, Zickert P, et al. Disruption of tubular Flcn expression as a mouse model for renal tumor induction. Kidney International. 2015;**88**(5):1057-1069

[28] Quddus MB, Pratt N, Nabi G. Chromosomal aberrations in renal cell carcinoma: An overview with implications for clinical practice. Urology Annals. 2019;**11**(1):6-14

[29] Chen J, Lui WO, Vos MD, Clark GJ, Takahashi M, Schoumans J, et al. The t(1;3) breakpoint-spanning genes LSAMP and NORE1 are involved in clear cell renal cell carcinomas. Cancer Cell. 2003;**4**(5):405-413

[30] Ohashi R, Schraml P, Angori S, Batavia AA, Rupp NJ, Ohe C, et al. Classic chromophobe renal cell carcinoma incur a larger number of chromosomal losses than seen in the eosinophilic subtype. Cancers (Basel). 2019;**11**(10):1492

[31] Tan MH, Wong CF, Tan HL, Yang XJ, Ditlev J, Matsuda D, et al. Genomic expression and single-nucleotide polymorphism profiling discriminates chromophobe renal cell carcinoma and oncocytoma. BMC Cancer. 2010;**10**:196

[32] Tsui KH, Shvarts O, Smith RB, Figlin R, de Kernion JB, Belldegrun A. Renal cell carcinoma: prognostic significance of incidentally detected tumors. The Journal of Urology. 2000;**163**(2):426-430

[33] Mota M, Bezerra ROF, Garcia MRT. Practical approach to primary retroperitoneal masses in adults. Radiologia Brasileira. 2018;**51**(6):391-400

[34] Helenon O, Crosnier A, Verkarre V, Merran S, Mejean A, Correas JM. Simple and complex renal cysts in adults: classification system for renal cystic masses. Diagnostic and Interventional Imaging. 2018;**99**(4):189-218

[35] Agnello F, Albano D, Micci G, Di Buono G, Agrusa A, Salvaggio G, et al. CT and MR imaging of cystic renal lesions. Insights Into Imaging. 2020;**11**(1):5

[36] Johnson PT, Horton KM, Fishman EK. Optimizing detectability of renal pathology with MDCT: protocols, pearls, and pitfalls. AJR. American Journal of Roentgenology. 2010;**194**(4):1001-1012

[37] Kim JH, Sun HY, Hwang J, Hong SS, Cho YJ, Doo SW, et al. Diagnostic accuracy of contrast-enhanced computed tomography and contrast-enhanced magnetic resonance imaging of small renal masses in real practice: sensitivity and specificity according to subjective radiologic interpretation. World Journal of Surgical Oncology. 2016;**14**(1):260

[38] Farolfi A, Koschel S, Murphy DG, Fanti S. PET imaging in urology: a rapidly growing successful collaboration. Current Opinion in Urology. 2020;**30**(5):623-627

[39] Courcier J, de la Taille A, Nourieh M, Leguerney I, Lassau N. Ingels A: Carbonic anhydrase IX in renal cell carcinoma, implications for disease management. International Journal of Molecular Sciences. 2020;**21**(19):7146

[40] Hora M, Eret V, Travnicek I, Prochazkova K, Pitra T, Dolejsova O, et al. Surgical treatment of kidney tumors - contemporary trends in clinical practice. Central European Journal of Urology. 2016;**69**(4):341-346

[41] Campbell S, Uzzo RG, Allaf ME, Bass EB, Cadeddu JA, Chang A, et al. Renal mass and localized renal cancer: AUA guideline. The Journal of Urology. 2017;**198**(3):520-529

[42] Sebastia C, Corominas D, Musquera M, Pano B, Ajami T, Nicolau C. Active surveillance of small renal masses. Insights Into Imaging. 2020;**11**(1):63

[43] Potretzke AM, Weaver J, Benway BM. Review of robot-assisted partial nephrectomy in modern practice. Journal of Kidney Cancer and VHL. 2015;**2**(2):30-44

[44] Phung MC, Lee BR. Recent advancements of robotic surgery for kidney cancer. Asian Journal of Endoscopic Surgery. 2018;**11**(4):300-307

[45] Ghani KR, Sukumar S, Sammon JD, Rogers CG, Trinh QD, Menon M. Practice patterns and outcomes of open and minimally invasive partial nephrectomy since the introduction of robotic partial nephrectomy: results from the nationwide inpatient sample. The Journal of Urology. 2014;**191**(4):907-912

[46] Li M, Cheng L, Zhang H, Ma L, Wang Y, Niu W, et al. Laparoscopic and robotic-assisted partial nephrectomy: an overview of hot issues. Urologia Internationalis. 2020;**104**(9-10):669-677

[47] Ljungberg B, Bensalah K, Canfield S, Dabestani S, Hofmann F, Hora M, et al.

EAU guidelines on renal cell carcinoma: 2014 update. European Urology. 2015;**67**(5):913-924

[48] Suek T, Davaro F, Raza SJ, Hamilton Z. Robotic surgery for cT2 kidney cancer: analysis of the National Cancer Database. Journal of Robotic Surgery. 2022;**16**(3):723-729

[49] Carbonara U, Amparore D, Borregales LD, Calio A, Ciccarese C, Diana P, et al. Single-port robotic partial nephrectomy: impact on perioperative outcomes and hospital stay. Therapeutic Advances in Urology. 2023;**15**:17562872231172834

[50] Salkowski M, Checcucci E, Chow AK, Rogers CC, Adbollah F, Liatsikos E, et al. New multiport robotic surgical systems: a comprehensive literature review of clinical outcomes in urology. Therapeutic Advances in Urology. 2023;**15**:17562872231177781

[51] Valero R, Sawczyn G, Garisto J, Yau R, Kaouk J. Multiquadrant combined robotic radical prostatectomy and left partial nephrectomy: a combined procedure by a single approach. Actas Urológicas Españolas (English Edition). 2020;**44**(2):119-124

[52] McDermott DF, Regan MM, Clark JI, Flaherty LE, Weiss GR, Logan TF, et al. Randomized phase III trial of high-dose interleukin-2 versus subcutaneous interleukin-2 and interferon in patients with metastatic renal cell carcinoma. Journal of Clinical Oncology. 2005;**23**(1):133-141

[53] Dizman N, Philip EJ, Pal SK. Genomic profiling in renal cell carcinoma. Nature Reviews. Nephrology. 2020;**16**(8):435-451

[54] Osawa T, Takeuchi A, Kojima T, Shinohara N, Eto M, Nishiyama H. Overview of current and future systemic therapy for metastatic renal cell carcinoma. Japanese Journal of Clinical Oncology. 2019;**49**(5):395-403

[55] Choueiri TK, Escudier B, Powles T, Mainwaring PN, Rini BI, Donskov F, et al. Cabozantinib versus everolimus in advanced renal-cell carcinoma. The New England Journal of Medicine. 2015;**373**(19):1814-1823

[56] Motzer RJ, Hutson TE, Glen H, Michaelson MD, Molina A, Eisen T, et al. Lenvatinib, everolimus, and the combination in patients with metastatic renal cell carcinoma: a randomised, phase 2, open-label, multicentre trial. The Lancet Oncology. 2015;**16**(15):1473-1482

[57] Motzer RJ, Escudier B, McDermott DF, George S, Hammers HJ, Srinivas S, et al. Nivolumab versus everolimus in advanced renal-cell carcinoma. The New England Journal of Medicine. 2015;**373**(19):1803-1813

[58] Jonasch E. NCCN guidelines updates: management of metastatic kidney cancer. Journal of the National Comprehensive Cancer Network. 2019;**17**(5.5):587-589

[59] Motzer RJ, Penkov K, Haanen J, Rini B, Albiges L, Campbell MT, et al. Avelumab plus axitinib versus sunitinib for advanced renal-cell carcinoma. The New England Journal of Medicine. 2019;**380**(12):1103-1115

[60] Rini BI, Plimack ER, Stus V, Gafanov R, Hawkins R, Nosov D, et al. Pembrolizumab plus axitinib versus sunitinib for advanced renal-cell carcinoma. The New England Journal of Medicine. 2019;**380**(12):1116-1127

[61] Angulo JC, Manini C, Lopez JI, Pueyo A, Colas B, Ropero S. The role of epigenetics in the progression of clear

cell renal cell carcinoma and the basis for future epigenetic treatments. Cancers (Basel). 2021;**13**(9):2071

[62] Xie L, Wu S, He R, Li S, Lai X, Wang Z. Identification of epigenetic dysregulation gene markers and immune landscape in kidney renal clear cell carcinoma by comprehensive genomic analysis. Frontiers in Immunology. 2022;**13**:901662

[63] Burlibasa L, Nicu AT, Chifiriuc MC, Medar C, Petrescu A, Jinga V, et al. H3 histone methylation landscape in male urogenital cancers: from molecular mechanisms to epigenetic biomarkers and therapeutic targets. Frontiers in Cell and Development Biology. 2023;**11**:1181764

[64] El Khoury LY, Fu S, Hlady RA, Wagner RT, Wang L, Eckel-Passow JE, et al. Identification of DNA methylation signatures associated with poor outcome in lower-risk Stage, Size, Grade and Necrosis (SSIGN) score clear cell renal cell cancer. Clinical Epigenetics. 2021;**13**(1):12

Chapter 2

Oncometabolite L-2-Hydroxyglutarate Promotes Oncogenesis of Renal Cell Carcinomas by Down-Regulating Differentiation

Mary Taub

Abstract

L-2-Hydroxyglutarate (L2HG) overproducing Renal Cell Carcinomas (RCCs) arise in the kidney due to the genetic loss of L-2HG Dehydrogenase (L2HGDH), the enzyme responsible for the metabolism of L2HG. The overproduced 2-Hydroxyglutarate (2HG) promotes tumorigenesis by inhibiting α-ketoglutarate (αKG)-dependent dioxygenases, including Ten-eleven-Translocation 5-methylcytosine (5mC) dioxygenase (TET) enzymes as well as histone demethylases. The resulting epigenetic changes alter the phenotype of renal proximal tubule (RPT) cells, the cells of origin of RCCs. This report describes the consequences of increased L2HG on the differentiation of RPT cells, one of the initial steps in promoting tumorigenesis. Presumably, similar alterations promote the expansion of renal cancer stem-cells and tumorigenesis.

Keywords: oncometabolite, L-2-Hydroxyglutarate, renal cell carcinoma, renal proximal tubule, epigenetic, tubulogenesis, dedifferentiation, matrigel

1. Introduction

Oncometabolites are components of intermediary metabolism whose abundance increases dramatically during the metabolic rewiring that occurs during tumorigenesis. These oncometabolites act to promote, and/or sustain tumor growth and metastasis. The hypothesis that metabolic rewiring plays a major role in tumorigenesis was initially supported by the work of Warburg in the 1920s. Warburg's experimental results indicated that aerobic glycolysis becomes the predominant means of generating the metabolic demands of developing tumors, rather than oxidative metabolism [1]. In recent years, the Warburg effect has been substantiated in studies of Clear Cell RCCs (ccRCCs) with von Hippel-Lindau (VHL) mutations, in addition to studies with other tumors [1]. In these tumors, aerobic glycolysis predominates over the tricarboxylic acid cycle (TCA) and oxidative phosphorylation. As a consequence, these tumor cells use glucose more efficiently than normal cells, producing lactic acid. The lactic acid is used as an alternative source of acetyl-Coenzyme A (acetyl-CoA) for the production of fatty acids and cholesterol [2]. Glutamine, is another essential component for the production of fatty acids and the lipid droplets characteristic of ccRCCs [2]. Following its entry into the mitochondria, glutamine (Gln) is converted to glutamate (Glu) by glutaminase, followed by conversion to αKG, which as we will see, is not only an important intermediate in the TCA cycle, but is also a precursor for the oncometabolite 2HG.

Numerous investigations have shown that the Warburg effect arises due to major changes in the expression of a number of glycolytic and TCA cycle enzymes [3]. In the majority of ccRCCs, both alleles of the von Hippel-Lindau (VHL) gene are mutated, leading to dysregulation of Hypoxia-inducible factor 1 (HIF-1) transcriptional activity. HIF-1, a master regulator of oxygen homeostasis, is hydroxylated on its α subunit during normoxia by a ubiquitin protein ligase, whose activity depends upon VHL. In the absence of normal VHL, HIF-1 reprograms glucose and energy metabolism through its transcriptional activities, such that glycolysis and lactate production become predominant over respiration, even during normoxia [3].

More recent studies indicate that mutations which specifically effect the expression of 3 different types of metabolic enzymes (fumarate hydratase (FH), succinate dehydrogenase (SDH) and isocitrate dehydrogenase (IDH)) similarly promote tumorigenesis because of the accumulation of "oncometabolites" [1]. Oncometabolites are defined as "small-molecule components (or enantiomers) of normal metabolism whose accumulation dysregulates signaling so as to establish a milieu that promotes carcinogenesis" [4]. The fumarate accumulation, which occurs as a consequence of FH mutations, results in the formation of hereditary papillary renal carcinomas, whereas the succinate accumulation, that occurs as a consequence of SDH mutations, results in the formation of hereditary paragangliomas (PGLs). In contrast, cancer-related mutations in the *IDH1* and *IDH2* genes, result in the formation of mutant IDH enzymes which produce D-2-hydroxyglutarate (D2HG) from αKG. This is particularly serious, because IDH1 and IDH2 mutations are associated with 70–80% glioblastomas, and 20% of acute myeloid leukemias (AMLs) [5]. All 3 oncometabolites, D2HG, fumarate and succinate, have been found to act by similar mechanisms, i.e. by inhibiting multiple αKG-dependent dioxygenases, which ultimately dysregulates signaling in a manner that promotes tumorigenesis [1, 5].

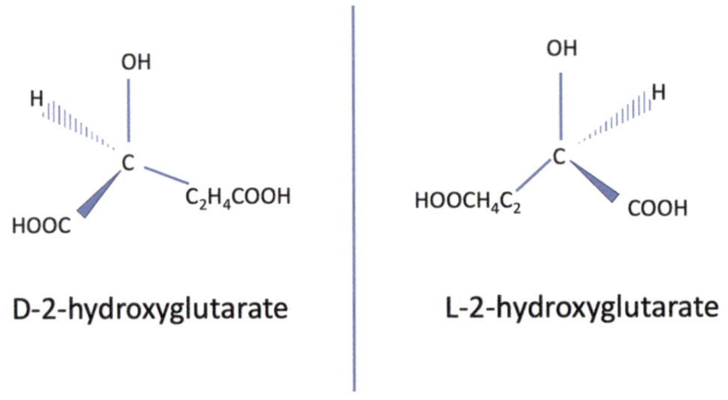

Figure 1.
The D- and L- enantiomers of L-2Hydroxglutarate (L-2HG).2HG is a chiral molecule, with D-and L-enantiomers as illustrated above.

Notably, oncometabolites such as 2HG have also been used as prognostic markers. In individuals with cancer-related IDH mutations, D2HG is produced to such an extent, that the elevated D2HG can be detected in serum [6]. Remarkedly, 87% of the AML patients with high serum 2HG had IDH1/IDH2 mutations, although only 29% of AML patients with moderately high 2HG had IDH1/IDH2 mutations. This latter finding suggests that other genetic events are also responsible for elevated 2HG. Of particular interest in these regards, 2HG is a chiral molecule, with both D- and L- enantiomers (as show in **Figure 1**). Both IDH1 and IDH2 mutations result in increased synthesis of the D- enantiomer (as shown in **Figure 2**). However, a loss of copy number of L2HGDH results in increased levels of the L- enantiomer of 2HG, rather than the D- enantiomer. For this reason, Struys [7] has stressed the importance of employing analytical methods that differentiate between L2HG and D2HG (e.g. chiral derivatization followed by Liquid Chromatography-Mass Spectrometry/Mass Spectrometry (LC–MS/MS)), rather than measuring total 2HG.

During the initial time frame of the studies in which elevated 2HG was detected in serum, an inherited metabolic defect, L-2-Hydroxyglutarate aciduria (L2HGA) was being studied [8]. L2HGA is an autosomal recessive neurometabolic disorder, characterized by abnormalities of the subcortical cerebral white matter dentate nucleus, globus pallidus, putamen and caudate nucleus. The gene associated with this disorder was found to be a mutant *L2HGDH*, which was defective in metabolizing L2HG to αKG. Consistent with this observation, the biochemical hallmark of L2HGA is elevated levels of L2HG in the urine (such that L2HG levels are 10–300 fold more than normal controls). A consequence of L2HGA is an increased propensity for tumor formation. Kranendijk et al. [8] have reported that L2HG is produced from αKG by L-malate dehydrogenase (MDH), as a promiscuous side reaction (**Figure 3**). The primary

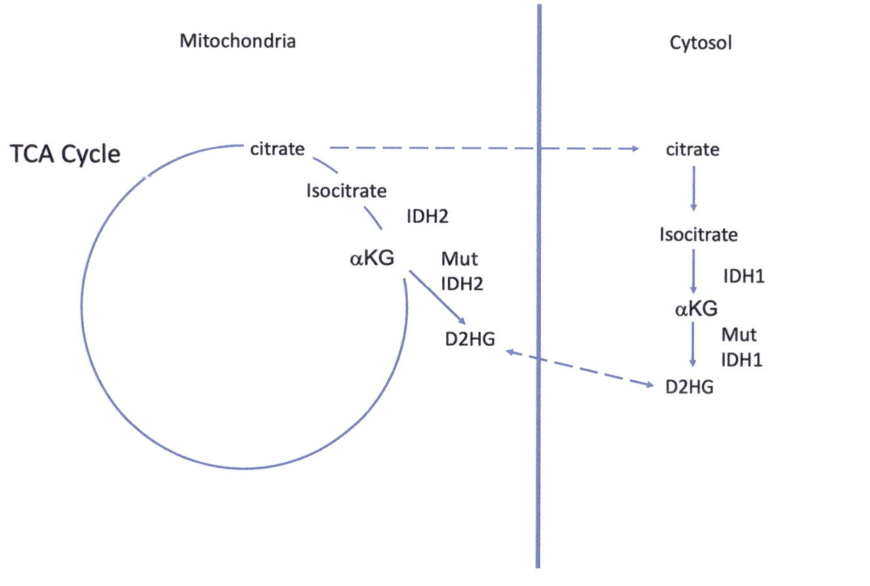

Figure 2.
Effect of mutant Isocitrate dehydrogenase (IDH) on metabolism of D-2HG. Two different isoforms of IDH are present in mammalian cells, including cytosolic IDH_1 and mitochondrial IDH_2, which participated in the tricarboxylic acid (TCA) cycle. Normally, IDH_1 or IDH_2 have been found to synthesize alpha ketoglutarate from isocitrate. However, mutant IDH_1 and IDH_2 have been found to further synthesize D-2HG from alpha ketogutarate.

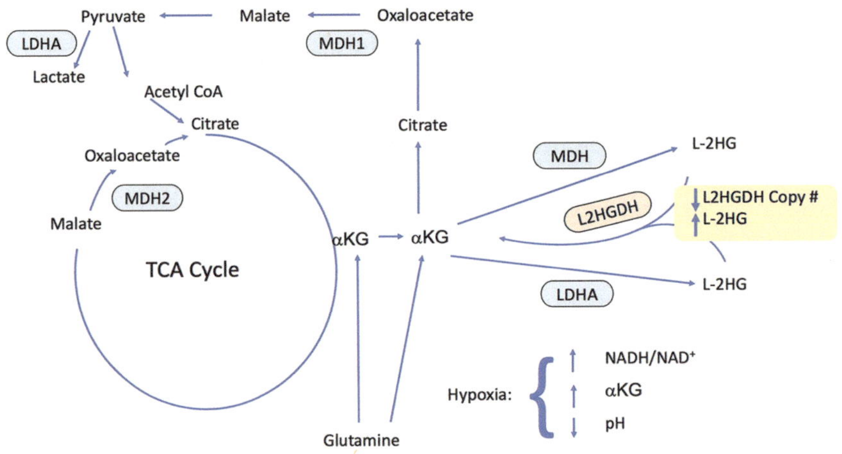

Figure 3.
Biosynthesis of L2HG from glutamine: Effect of a loss of L2HGDH copy number. The biosynthesis of L2HG depends upon glutamine (Gln), which is first metabolized to glutamine acid by Glutaminase, followed by the metabolism of alpha ketoglutarate. Alpha ketoglutarate generated either by the TCA cycle or in mitochondria or in the cytosol, is subsequently metabolized by either malate dehydrogenase (MDH) or by lactate dehydrogenase a (LDHA) into L2HG. When the copy number of L2HG Deydrogenase (L2HGDH) declines, the metabolism of L2HG slows, causing an increase in the level of L2HG.

function of MDH is to convert L-malate to oxaloacetate. Lactate Dehydrogenase (LDH) has similarly been found to produce L2HG as a side reaction during oxygen deprivation under acidic conditions (**Figure 3**) [9]. In contrast, D2HG is produced from γ hydroxybutyrate by hydroxyacid-oxoacid transhydrogenase (HOT) [8].

As stated above, patients with L2HGA exhibit neurological disorders, associated with progressive damage to the brain. Biochemical alterations in brain tissues include reduced creatine kinase activity, oxidative stress, and increased Glutamate (Glu) uptake into synaptosomes and synaptic vesicles. Precisely why the brain is primarily affected is not well understood.

Subsequent to the findings that the D2HG enantiomer is elevated in glioblastomas and AMLs, other investigators found that other enantiomer, L2HG, is indeed elevated in another class of tumors, ccRCCs [10]. The elevated L2HG has been attributed to a loss of copies of the L2HGDH gene [11], encoding for the enzyme that metabolizes L2HG to αKG [10]. Elevated L2HG and reduced L2HGDH was observed in a number of human RCC cell lines, including A498, RXF-393 and Caki-1, and in addition was a common attribute of ccRCCs obtained from patients [10]. In order to determine whether the decreased L2HGDH contributes to tumorigenicity, A498 cells were transduced with a WT L2HGDH vector (generating A498-L2HGD). Not only were the L2HG levels reduced in A498-L2HGDH cells, but the volume of A498-L2HGDH tumors was reduced, as compared with controls [10]. L2HG levels are determined by its biosynthetic rate, as well as by its degradation. Shelar et al. [11] reported that L2HG in RCC cells is generated from αKG by MDH1 and MDH2, via promiscuous reactions.

2. Epigenetic effects of L- and D-2HG

Both L2HG and D2HG are competitive inhibitors of αKG-dependent dioxygenases. The specific αKG-dependent dioxygenase(s) which are the targets of elevated L2HG in the brain of patients with L2HGA has not yet been identified. However, the most notable known targets of L2HG and D2HG in tumors are epigenetic targets, including αKG-dependent dioxygenases that regulate either DNA or histone demethylation. Included amongst these αKG-dependent dioxygenases that are inhibited by L2HG and D2HG are Jumonji domain-containing histone-lysine demethylases (Jmj-KDMs), that demethylate histones, as well as TETs, which demethylate 5-methyl-cytosine (5mC) residues in genomic DNA. Consequences of the inhibition of these dioxygenases by L2HG and D2HG include the increased methylation of histone marks, as well as an increase in 5mC residues in CpG islands [12]. While both enantiomers of 2HG inhibit Jmj-KDMs as well as TETs, overall L2HG is a more potent inhibitor than D2HG [13].

The Jmj-KDMs demethylate lysine residues on specific classes of methylated histones, their specificity being determined by specific reader domains present within each type of protein [14]. For example, JmjD2A and JmD3 remove a methyl group from the repressive histones H3K9me3, and H3K27me3, respectively, whereas JARID1A removes a methyl group from the activating histone H3K4me3 (**Table 1**) [14]. In this manner the Jmj-KDMs reverse the methylation events caused by corresponding Histone Lysine Methyltransferases (abbreviated as either KMTs or HMTs) (**Table 1**) [15].

The TETs demethylate 5mC residues in genomic DNA in a number of steps. Initially, TETs oxidize 5mC, generating 5-hydroxy-mC (5hmC), followed by further oxidation of 5hmC into 5-formylcytosine (5fC), and finally 5-carboxycytosine (5caC). Subsequently, the modified base is removed, and excision repair occurs [16]. Point mutations and deletion mutations are often observed in human cancers, particularly those affecting TET2 (as observed in AML). This latter observation is consistent with the hypothesis that the inactivation of TETs by D2HG plays a similar role in AML [16].

In their studies, Chowdhury et al. [13] found that 2HG is a weak antagonist of αKG (requiring a 100-fold molar excess of 2HG over αKG). This molar excess of 2HG can nevertheless be achieved in cells with IDH mutations. The concentration of D2HG increases to as high as 35 mM in cells with IDH mutations, exceeding the IC50 of 2HG for Jmj-KDMs [13]. In such IDH mutant cells, αKG is itself consumed, being the substrate of 2HG, further increasing the inhibition by 2HG. Although the evidence is convincing that D2HG and L2HG alter the epigenetic landscape in cells, inhibitory effects of 2HG on other classes of αKG-dependent dioxygenases, may also promote tumorigenesis. For example, L2HG inhibits Prolyl Hydroxylase 2 (PHD2), thereby preventing the hydroxylation of HIF1α, and the degradation of HIF1α by the

	H3K9me2/3	**H3K27me2/3**	**H3K4me2/3**	**H3K36me3**
KMT	G9a/EHMT2	EZH1	SETD1A	SETD2
KMT	GLP/EHMT1	EZH2	SETD1B	NSD1
Jmj-KDM	JmjD2A (KDM4A)	JmjD3 (KDM6B)	JARID1A	JmjD2A (KDM4A)
Jmj-KDM	JmjD2C (KDM4C)	UTX (KDM6A)	JARID1B	JmjD2B (KDM4B)

Methylated Histones are listed in the top row, which have been methylated by the histone lysine methyltransferases (KMTs) in the first 2 rows listed directly below the particular KMT. In the third and fourth rows are listed the histone demethylases (in particular the Jmj-KDMs) which demethylate the histones listed in the same column as the particular Jm-KDMs.

Table 1.
Representative histone lysine Methyltransferases (KMTs), with associated Jmj-KDMs and histone substrates.

proteosome [9]. Collagen hydroxylase is also inhibited by L2HG and D2HG, which perturbs basement membrane function [17]. Finally, D2HG and L2HG inhibit the repair of DNA alkylating damage (via ALK Homolog, i.e. ALKBH, enzymes), which promotes oncogenesis [17].

3. Effects of D-2HG on adipocyte and myocyte differentiation

Of particular interest to this review are the L2HG mediated effects on renal differentiation, so as to increase the propensity of renal cells to become tumorigenic. However, previous studies concerning the effects of D2HG on the differentiation of other cell types will first be described, to facilitate our understanding of effects of L2HG on renal differentiation, including epigenetic changes. Both D2HG and L2HG inhibit αKG-dependent dioxygenases, although admittedly the 2 enantiomers have different binding affinities for a number of αKG-dependent dioxygenases. Nevertheless, previous studies of the effects of D2HG on differentiation in other tissues, will facilitate our understanding of how L2HG alters kidney development.

The effects of D2HG on differentiation were initially studied because gliomas with IDH mutations had a gene expression profile enriched for genes expressed in neural progenitor cells [18]. Moreover, increased levels of repressive H3K9me3 and H3K27me3 were observed in oligodendrogliomas with IDH1 mutations compared to tumors with wild type IDH1 [18]. Presumably, this was a consequence of the elevated D2HG in these tumors. Consistent with this hypothesis increased histone methylation was observed in 293 cells expressing a mutant IDH1 (or mutant IDH2) as compared to the wild type IDH allele.

In order to determine whether D2HG could block the differentiation of non-transformed cells, studies were conducted with 3T3-L1 cells which could be induced to differentiate into adipocytes using a differentiation cocktail [18]. 3T3-L1 cells transduced with an R172K mutant IDH2, overproduced D2HG, unlike cells transduced with WT IDH2 or empty vector. After induction of differentiation, the mutant IDH2 expressing 3T3-L1 cells had a markedly reduced ability to accumulate lipid droplets and were defective in the expression of transcription factors required for adipocyte differentiation, including CEBPA (CCAAT Enhancer Binding Protein α) and PPARγ (Peroxisome Proliferator-Activated Receptor γ, encoded by the *Pparg* gene). The impaired differentiation was associated with increased levels of H3K9me3 and H3K27me3. H3K9me3 in particular was located on the promoters of the *Cebpa* and *Pparg* genes. The increased H3K9me3 was attributed to the inhibition of the histone demethylase KDM4C by D2HG. Indeed, KDM4C was induced during the differentiation of 3T3L1 cells into adipocytes, and a knockdown of KDM4C with siRNA inhibited differentiation. Of particular interest in these regards KDM4C (which demethylates H3K9me3), is a member of the JHDM family of histone demethylases (i.e. JmjC domain-containing histone demethylases, or jmj-KDMs). Notably, H3K9me3 is the product of the G9a methyltransferase, which is known to produce repressive histones [14].

Subsequently, Schvartzman et al. [19] presented evidence indicating that the elevated D2HG (produced by oncogenic IDH1/2 mutations) similarly blocked the differentiation of 10T1/2 cell into myocytes by preventing H3K9 demethylation. Indeed, the HMT inhibitor UNC0638 (which blocks the H3K9 methylation by EHMT1/2) restored the ability of 10T1/2 cells expressing IDH2-R172K to form fused myotubes. Furthermore, similar results were obtained by a Clustered Regularly Interspaced

Short Palindromic Repeat (CRISPR) mediated deletion of EHMT1/2. The differentiation of 10T1/2 cells into myocytes depends upon the MyoD transcription factor. Very importantly, a Chromatin Immunoprecipitation Sequencing (ChIP-Seq) analysis indicated that the IDH2-R172K mutant did not have a global effect on chromatin accessibility in differentiating 10T1/2 cells. Instead, the IDH2-R172K mutant specifically prevented a MyoD-mediated increase in chromatin accessibility at myogenic regions. Thus, the authors conclude that the histone methylations that occur within genetic regions present within "facultative" heterochromatin are responsible for the 2HG-mediated block in differentiation, rather than random methylation events. Further studies of these 2HG-mediated blocks in differentiation, will reveal the precise nature of the 2HG-mediated genomic changes that contribute to tumorigenesis.

4. Effects of L2HG on ccRCCs

The transcriptional basis of nephron-specific gene expression patterns that emerge during nephrogenesis are incompletely understood. However, alterations in histone and DNA methylation caused by oncometabolites such as 2HG may very well upset the network of interactions established by transcription factors (TFs), so as to alter "normal" patterns of differentiated gene expression, and to cause "dedifferentiation." Nevertheless, Lindgren et al. [20] were able to identify remnants of cell type specific gene expression programs in a number of kidney cancers, and in this manner identify their lineage. Although many fundamental genetic alterations which contribute to the formation of RCCs have been identified, an understanding of the changes which occur in the specific cell subpopulation(s) that are the cells of origin of RCCs is nevertheless of importance. Lindgren et al. [20] were able to identify a gene cluster (cluster B) that was expressed in ccRCCs that corresponds with genes expressed in the renal proximal tubule (including trans-membrane transporters regulated by the Hepatocyte Nuclear Factor (HNF) TF family, most notably HNF4α which plays a role in RPT differentiation [21]). In addition, another gene cluster (cluster C) was over-expressed in ccRCCs (including genes regulated by HIF1α and expressed during hypoxia, angiogenesis as well as the epithelial-mesenchymal transition (EMT)). A number of the changes in gene cluster C are often associated the loss of VHL. In contrast, chromophobe RCCs expressed a Forkhead box protein L1 (FOXl1) gene signature. FOXI1 plays a critical role in the differentiation of intercalated cells in the connecting tubules and collecting ducts during renal development [22].

Although some remnants of normal transcription may remain, transcriptional changes that result in a loss of differentiation is a hallmark of many tumors. When considering ccRCCs in particular, evidence for changes in the activity of histone demethylases (including jmj-KDMs) has been obtained [23]. These changes alter the genetic landscape, resulting in the reduced expression of genes that encode for differentiated functions. Included amongst these genes, are genes encoding for renal transporters, proteins which maintain the polarized epithelial morphology, as well as proteins required for progression through the cell cycle, and apoptosis [24]. Gene silencing due to the hypermethylation of DNA and histones, is a strong candidate mechanism underlying the block in differentiation in ccRCCs. Of particular interest, is the role of elevated L2HG in such renal tumors, because increased L2HG is associated with increases in histone as well as DNA methylation. Indeed, Shelar et al. [11] observed increased H3K27 trimethylation in A498 RCC cells that have elevated levels of L2HG. In addition, there was a decrease in the expression of genes targeted by the

Polycomb Repressor Complex 2 (PRC2), including genes targeted by Suz12, that bear the H3K27me3 mark in human embryonic stem cells [11]. These results suggest there is an interrelationship between the changes in the gene expression profiles observed during embryonic development, and the gene expression changes caused by L2HG in renal carcinomas.

5. Epigenetic and transcriptional changes during renal development

Strikingly, during renal development, there is an interplay between the repressive effects of PRC2 proteins, and stimulatory effects of Trithorax proteins [25]. Repressive histones, including H3K9me2 and H3K27me3, are generated by PRC2 in the metanephric mesenchyme which surrounds the ureteric bud (which includes quiescent cells with low levels of the Six2 and Lhx1 transcription factors). As development proceeds, the mesenchyme condenses. The condensed mesenchyme becomes enriched with the activating histone H3K4me3, indicating it was poised for activation. Somewhat later, nascent nephrons emerge, which have high levels of H3K4me3 and low levels of repressive H3K9me3 and H3K27me3, activating such genes as Lhx1. After nascent nephron cells emerge, Notch2 appears, an important transcription factor in RPT development.

Of particular interest, are the developmental events that occur during segmentation of the nephron, because during this period Renal Proximal Tubules (RPTs) appear, RPTs being the cell of origin of ccRCCs and papillary RCCs [26, 27]. HNF TFs emerge during this developmental stage, including HNF4α, which facilitates the formation of H3K4me2 to maintain active chromatin during this developmental period [28]. HNF1α is similarly active during this developmental period, recruiting KDM6A (i.e. UTX), resulting in the demethylation of H3K27me3, thereby relieving polycomb repression [29]. In contrast, loss of HNF1α function (which has been observed in ccRCCs) [30] results in polycomb repression. A similar loss of HNF1α function has been reported in other cancers, including non-small cell lung cancers [31], oral squamous carcinomas [32], and pancreatic cancers [29]. In the case of pancreatic cancers, re-expression of HNF1α reactivated differentiated acinar cell programs, and in this manner suppressed the emergence of pancreatic cancers [29]. Presumably, there is a potential to similarly override 2HG mediated blocks in differentiation programs in other cancers, including RCCs, by re-establishing required regulation by HNFs. For this reason, an evaluation of the effects of elevated 2HG on the differentiation of renal cells is important, including effects of 2HG on such transcription factors as HNF1α.

6. Effects of L2HG on renal differentiation and development *in vitro*

L2HG mediated effects on the differentiation of RPT cells have been examined, utilizing a well characterized primary culture system of normal renal cells. Primary cultures of kidney epithelial cells derived from purified rabbit RPTs were grown in serum free medium, supplemented with 5 μg/ml human insulin, 5 μg/ml human transferrin and 5×10^{-8} M hydrocortisone. Epithelial monolayers formed with a polarized morphology, and membrane transport systems distinctive of the RPT, including an apical Na^+/glucose cotransport system (SGLT2), a Na^+/phosphate cotransport system (NPT2a), a Na^+/H^+ antiport system (NHE3), and a basolateral p-Amino Hippurate (pAH) transport system (i.e. OAT1) (**Figure 4**) [33, 34]. The

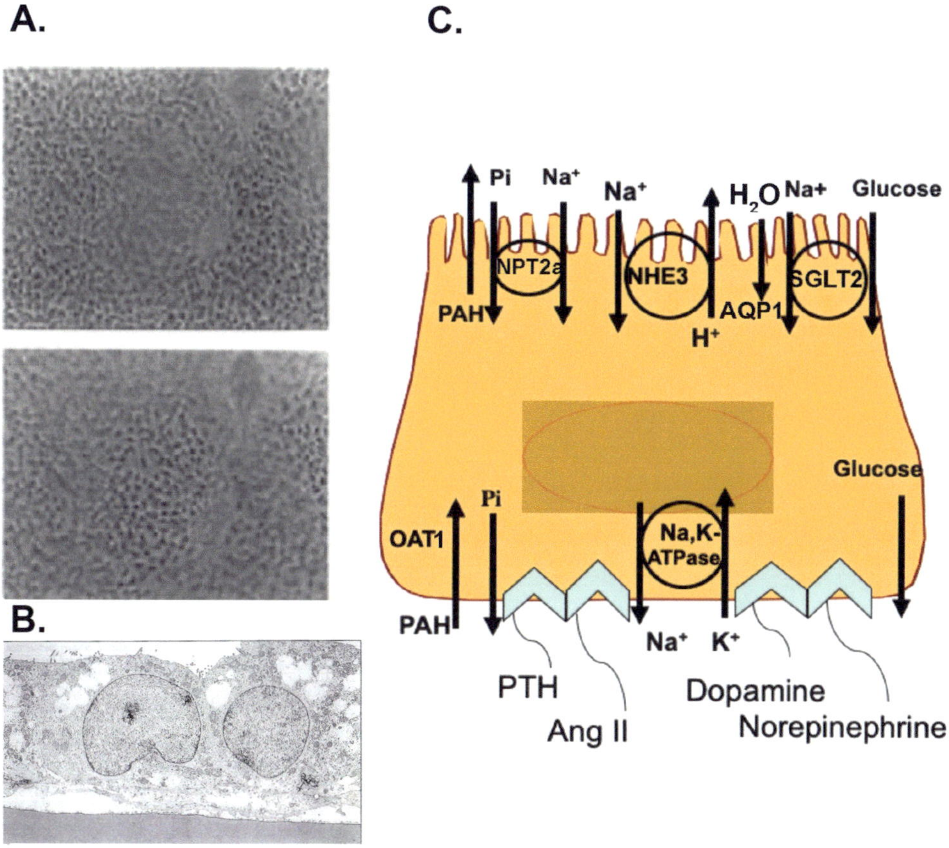

Figure 4.
Polarized morphology and transporters of primary proximal tubule (RPT) cells. A primary RPT cells form multicellular domes in culture. Groups of cells are elevated from the dish due to the accumulation of fluids between the monolayer and the dish, resulting from the transepithelial transport of fluids, and the resulting hydrostatic pressure. Two micrograoph fields are illustrated at t 100X. B. Transmission electron micrograph (TEM) of primary RPT cells. The TEM (illustrated at 2000X) shows the polarized morophology and interconnection of cells by tight junctions) from Taub et al. [34], reproduced with from Biotechniques, as agreed by future science, LTD) C. polarized transporters expressed in primary RPT cells as further defined in **Table 2.**

primary RPT cells also possess a parathyroid hormone (PTH) sensitive adenylate cyclase, Angiotensin II (Ang II) receptors [35], dopamine receptors, as well as α and β adrenergic receptors [36], which are critical for the regulation of ion transporters (**Figure 4**). Finally, the cultures retain normal metabolism, including gluconeogenesis, glutathione metabolism and other drug metabolic capabilities distinctive of the RPT (**Table 2**).

The effects of L2HG on primary RPT cells were examined both in 3-Dimensional (3D) matrigel cultures, as well as monolayer cultures. Such 3D culture systems are the method of choice for examining malignant cells *ex vivo* [37], including the effects of oncometabolites on differentiation (which relate to tumor progression). Matrigel, a reconstituted basement membrane from the Engelbreth-Holm-Swarm (EHS) tumor, is particularly important to use in 3D studies. Matrigel is a well-characterized 3D system used to study differentiation in both normal and malignant tissues [38]. Matrigel was initially employed to study baby mouse kidney epithelial cells *ex vivo*. Tubulogenesis was observed, provided that either Epidermal Growth Factor (EGF)

Brush Border Enzymes	Apical Membrane Transporters	Basolateral Membrane Transporters	Responses to Effectors	Metabolism
Alkaline Phosphatase	Na^+/glucose cotransporter: SGLT2	Organic Anion (OAT1; p-Amino-hippurate transporter)	Hormones: Insulin, Estrogen, Hydrocortisone, Parathyroid Hormone	Gluconeogenesis
γ Glutamyl Transpeptidase	Na^+/Pi cotransporter: NPT2a	Na,K-ATPase	Renal Effectors: Angiotensin II, Norepinephrine, Dopamine	Glutathione
Leucine Aminopeptidase	Na^+/H^+ antiporter: NHE3		Growth Factors: EGF, FGF, HGF	Responsiveness to Toxicants
	Aquaporin 1: AQP1			

Primary rabbit RPT cells are cultured in serum free medium supplemented with insulin, transferrin and hydrocortisone. The method for culturing the primary RPT cells and their extensive characterization has been described by Taub [33].

Table 2.
Characteristics of primary RPT cells in culture.

or Transforming Growth Factor α (TGFα) were added to the culture medium [39]. Electron micrographs indicated that the baby mouse kidney tubules resembled collecting ducts [39].

Subsequently, a 3D system of renal proximal tubulogenesis was developed, using primary rabbit RPT cells [40]. The primary RPT cells form tubules in matrigel (**Figure 5**). The tubules possess transepithelial transport capacity, as indicated by their ability to secrete lucifer yellow (an organic anion) into the luminal space of the tubules [41]. This was indicated by the green fluorescence observed in the lumen of lucifer yellow treated cultures in matrigel. Tubulogenesis by RPTs was stimulated by EGF (similar to baby mouse kidney cells), as well as Hepatocyte Growth Factor (HGF). Because the RPT is the cell of origin of ccRCCs, this primary RPT cell culture system is an appropriate model system to examine effects of oncometabolite L2HG on RPT differentiation.

As described above, the elevated L2HG detected in RCCs, has been attributed to decreased expression of L2HGDH, the enzyme that breaks down L2HG to αKG. The results of a microarray study indicate that the expression of genes targeted by the Polycomb protein Suz-12 was reduced in L2HGDH deficient ccRCC cells, similar to the metanephric mesenchyme [42]. Thus, the hypothesis was examined, that reduced expression of L2HGDH blocks differentiation of renal cells.

In order to examine this hypothesis initially, primary RPT cell cultures were transduced with lentiviral particles containing a vector (pLKO-TRC) encoding either L2HGDH shRNA or control shRNA [43]. The effect on tubulogenesis in matrigel was examined. **Figure 6** shows the lack of tubules in cultures treated with L2HGDH shRNA, under conditions where L2HGDH mRNA was reduced by 80%. Tubulogenesis was similarly inhibited in primary RPT cells using L2HGDH siRNA, which similarly reduced L2HGDH mRNA by 80%. The effect of L2HGDH siRNA on intracellular L2HG and D2HG levels was examined by Gas Chromatography–Mass Spectrometry (GC–MS) analysis. The L2HG level increased more than 4-fold in

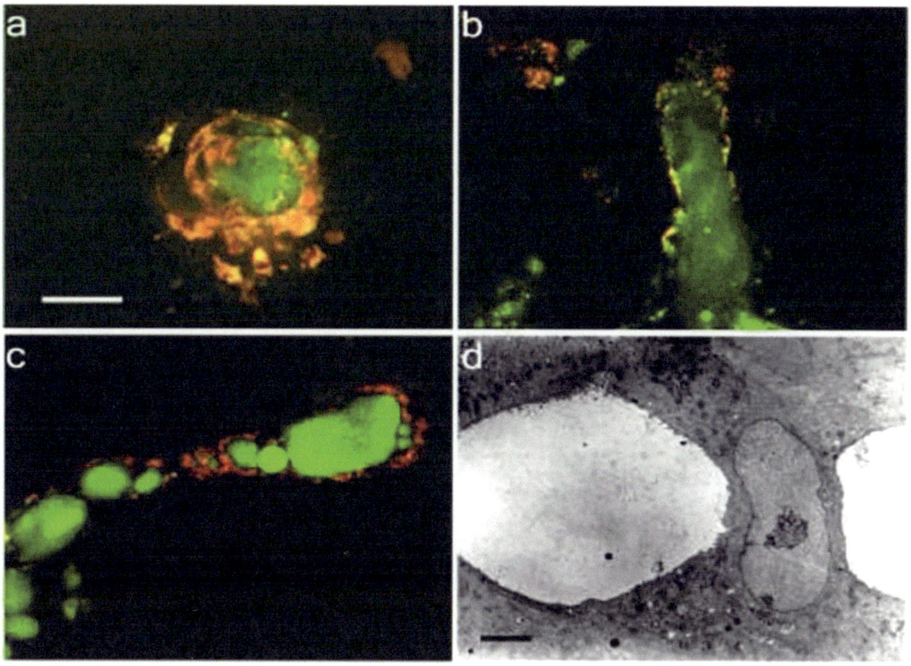

Figure 5.
Tubule formation by primary PRT cells in Matrigel. A. Traverse section of a tubule. Lucifer yellow accumulation (green) in the lumen of a tubule in matrigel, with DIl (yellow), a membrane stain. B. Longitudinal section of another tubule, C. section of developing tubule. D Cross-section of a tubule examined by TEM showing a lumen (L), and a nucleus (N). Bar is 50 μM in a, B and C. Bar in D is 10 μm. From Han et al. [41] with permission from the Company of Biologists.

primary RPTs treated with L2HGDH siRNA, L2HG becoming the predominant enantiomer.

Shelar et al. [11] observed that L2HG is primarily generated from Glutamine (Gln) in human ccRCCs, initially via the breakdown of Gln to Glu by glutaminase (as illustrated in **Figure 3**). Thus, the inhibition of Gln metabolism to Glu by glutaminase would be expected to reduce the L2HG level, and in this manner overcome the effect of an L2HGDH Knockdown (KD) on intracellular L2HG levels. In order to examine this hypothesis, the ability of primary RPT cells with an L2HGDH KD to form tubules in the presence of glutaminase inhibitor CB-839 was examined. The results (illustrated in **Figure 7**) indicated that CB-839 relieved the inhibition of tubulogenesis caused by an L2HGDH KD, presumably by reducing L2HG levels (a consequence of inhibiting the metabolism of Gln to Glu, and ultimately to L2HG). The involvement of the elevated L2HG in mediating the inhibition of tubulogenesis in cultures with an L2HGDH KD was further substantiated by the observed inhibitory effect of cell permeable L2HG octyl ester on tubulogenesis [43].

The block in tubulogenesis in primary RPT cells with an L2HGDH KD may very well be associated with a generalized loss of differentiated function. Consistent with this hypothesis, the expression of differentiated transporters was reduced in the primary RPT cells with an L2HGDH KD. This is exemplified by the reduction in the mRNA levels for the apical Na^+/Phosphate cotransporter (NPT2a), the Na^+/glucose cotransporter (SGLT2), and Aquaporin 1 (AQP1), as well as the basolateral pAH transporter (OAT1) in monolayers with an L2HGDH KD.

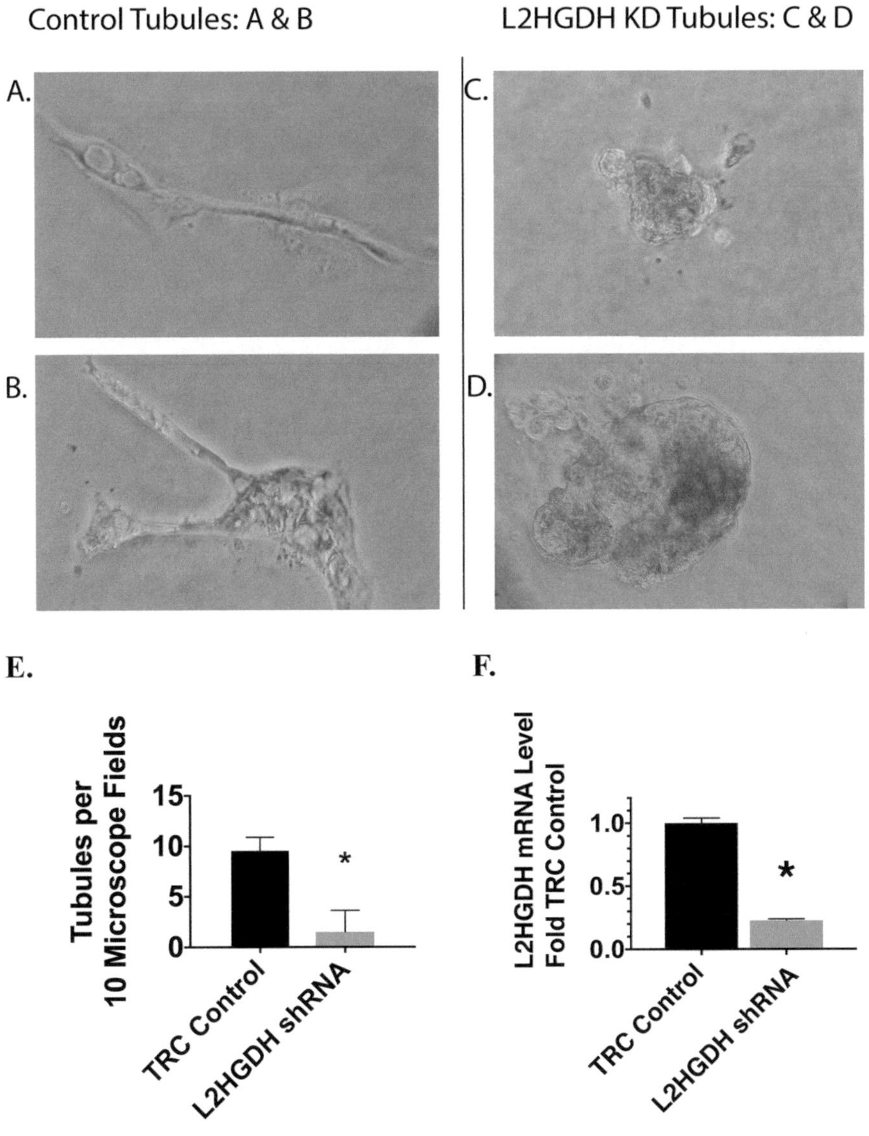

Figure 6.
Effect of L2HGDH shRNA on Tubulogenesis, primary RPT cells cultures were transduced with lentivirus containing either L2HGDH shRNA or control TRC shRNA vectors. The cultures put into matrigel. Subsequently, tubules photographed (A, B, C, D) at 100X. Tubules were quantitated and L2HGDH mRNA level were determined. From Taub et al. [43] with permission of Frontiers.

In matrigel cultures, the level of expression of NPT2a and SGLT2 increased relative to plastic in control cultures, consistent with the hypothesis that the overall state of differentiation was enhanced in matrigel. Nevertheless, the expression of these 2 transporters continued to be substantially reduced in cultures with an L2HGDH KD. In contrast, AQP1 expression increased in matrigel cultures with an L2HGDH KD. This observation can be explained by differences in transcriptional regulation between NPT2a and SGLT2 as compared with AQP1. Both NPT2a and SGLT2 regulation depends upon HNF1α which is down regulated in primary RPT cells with an

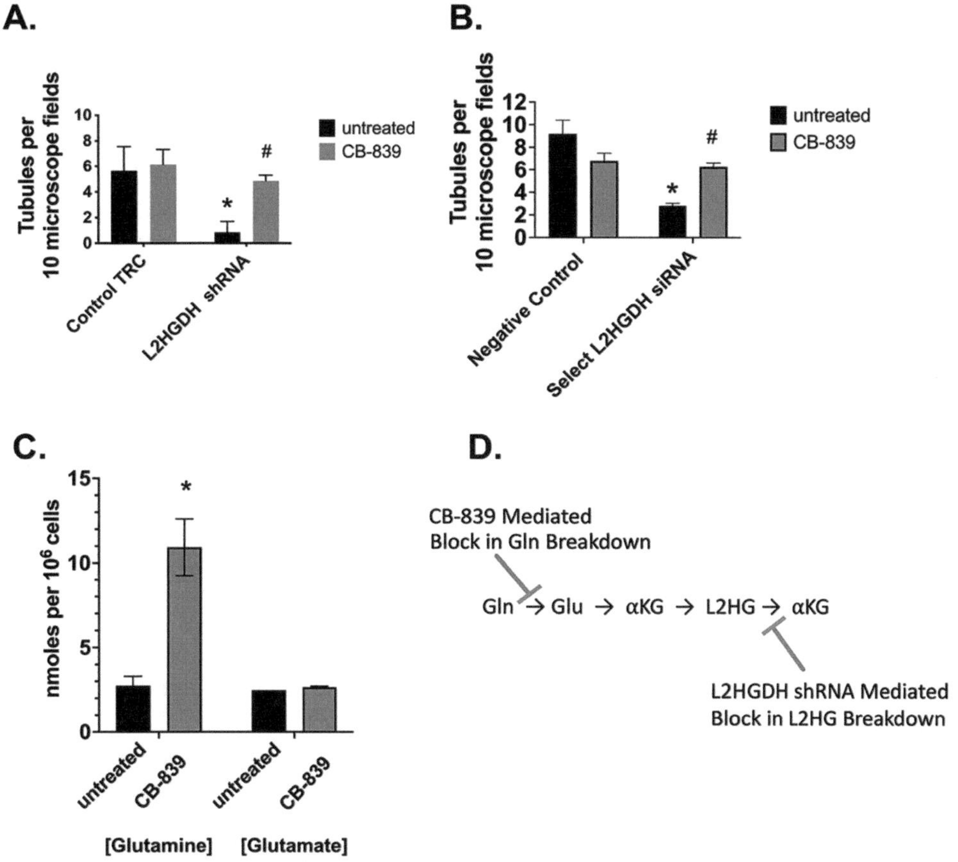

Figure 7.
Effect of Glutaminase inhibitor CB-839 on tubulogenesis. A. Primary RPT cells were either a. transduced with lentivirus containing either L2HGDH shRNA or control TRC shRNA vectors, or B. transfected with L2HGDH shRNA or negative control siRNA. The cultures were passaged into matrigel, and treated with either with 1 μM CB-839 or untreated. Subsequently, the frequency of tubule formation was determined [41]. C. the effect of 1 μM CB-839 on the level of glutamine and glutamate was determined [41]. D. Model for the effect of CB-839 on L2HGDH levels. Values are averages (+/−) SEMs of triplicate determinations. With permission from Frontiers.

L2HGDH KD, unlike AQP1, whose transcription is controlled by Tonicity Enhancer Binding Protein (TonEBP) and HIF1α. As described above, HNF1α is involved in the appearance of RPTs during kidney development. Thus, it will be of interest to determine whether during tubulogenesis in vitro, HNF1A recruits KDM6A, which relieves polycomb repression during this stage of kidney development by demethylating H3K27me3.

HNF1α has also been reported to play a role in maintaining the polarized morphology of epithelial cells. Indeed, inhibition of HNF1α gene expression with siRNA triggered the Epithelial to Mesenchymal Transition (EMT) in the liver cancer cell lines HEPG2 and HEP1B [44]. The expression of mRNAs encoding for such proteins as E-cadherin (CDH1) and plasminogen activator (PLAU) was similarly reduced in primary RPTs with an L2HGDH KD, as well as cell migration. Further studies are necessary to elucidate whether the downregulation of HNF1α under these conditions is responsible for these changes.

The downregulation of the expression of the differentiated transporters, and HNF1α in primary RPT cells with an L2HGDH KD is presumably a consequence of the inhibition of αKG dependent dioxygenases. Included amongst these αKG dependent dioxygenases are Jmj-KDM histone demethylases, as well as TET 5mC demethylases, which are inhibited not only in tumor cells with IDH1 and IDH2 mutations [45], but also in ccRCCs with reduced L2HGDH levels [11]. Consistent with this hypothesis, 5hmC blots of genomic DNA derived from primary RPT cells with an L2HGDH KD indicated that the level of 5hmC was reduced in primary RPT cells with an L2HGDH KD (vs. controls) [43]. In addition, Western blots indicated increases in the levels of a number of different classes of methylated histones in primary RPT cells with an L2HGD KD [43]. Not only was there an increase in the level of the activating histone, H3K4me3, but also an increase in the level of the repressive histone H3K27me3. Shelar et al. [11] similarly observed an increased level of H3K27me3 in A498 ccRCC cells as compared to A498 ccRCC cells which express exogenous L2HGDH. H3K27me3 is generated by EZH2, a component of the repressive PRC2 complex expressed in the primitive mesenchyme.

However, as described above, Schvartzman et al. [19] reported that the inhibitory effect of D2HG on the MyoD-mediated differentiation of myocytes was the specific consequence of increased H3K9 methylation generated by EHMT1/2. Schvartzman et al. [19] found that 5mC DNA hypermethylation could be excluded from in the differentiation block in 10 T1/2 cells, because the DNA methyltransferase inhibitor 5-azacytidine was unable to rescue the differentiation block caused by elevated D-2HG. The hypothesis that the inhibition of renal proximal tubulogenesis is similarly the specific consequence of increased H3K9 methylation cannot be excluded, in the absence of results with H3K9me3.

However, L2HG does not necessarily act on renal differentiation via the same mechanism as observed with D2HG in myocytes. Indeed, L2HG has a higher affinity than D2HG for a number of αKG-dependent dioxygenases, including TET 5hmC hydroxylases [45]. Furthermore, L2HG (unlike D2HG) is an effective inhibitor of such αKG dioxygenases as Prolyl Hydroxylase 2 (PDH2) (which promotes the degradation of HIF1α during normoxia) [17]. The effects of L2HG on other aspects of basic metabolism have not been extensively investigated. Thus, it is unclear whether L2HG, like D2HG causes a reduction in Nicotine Adenine Dinucleotide (NAD^+) levels, associated with a reduction in the level of Naprt (Nicotinate Phosphoribosyltransferase), a rate limiting enzyme in the NAD^+ salvage pathway that replenishes intracellular NAD^+ levels [46]. In any case, the effects of L2HG on differentiation of RPT cells ultimately depend upon the unique sets of epigenetic mechanisms that regulate kidney development, unlike other tissues.

Nevertheless, the L2HG-mediated inhibition of kidney proximal tubulogenesis very likely results at least in part from the inhibition of Jmj-KDMs. Previous studies indicate that histone demethylases, as well as histone methyltransferases play an important role in kidney development. It is well-known, as stated above, that during kidney development there is an interplay between events mediated by repressive PRC2 and stimulatory Trithorax complexes [25]. Different classes of methylated histones are produced by these 2 sets of complexes. While the histone methyltransferase Ash21 (associated with Trithorax complexes) produces activating H3K4me histones, Ezh1, Ezh2 and Suz12 (associated with PRC2) produce repressive H3K9me2/3 and H3K27me3. During the segmentation of the nephron, H3K4me histone levels increase as proximal tubules appear, while H3K9me2/3 and H3K27me3 levels decline. Remarkably, an increase in the level of both H3K9me3 and H3K27me3 is associated with the block in the ability of 10T1/2 cells with a mutant IDH2-R172K to differentiate into myocytes.

A decline in H3K9me2/3 and H3K27me3 during kidney development depends not only upon the activity of the pertinent histone methyltransferases, but also upon the continued activity of pertinent JmjC domain containing histone demethylases. While KDM4A, B, C and D demethylate H3K9me3, the transcriptionally activating KDM7A demethylates H3K9me1/2. Similarly, the demethylation H3K27me3 involves KDM4D, as well as KDM7A. However, given that these KDMs are αKG dependent dioxygenases, they are subject to inhibition by elevated D- and L-2HG. In the case of 10T1/2 cells expressing a mutant IDH enzyme, inhibition of KDM4C (which normally demethylates H3K9me3) was proposed to be responsible for their inability to differentiate into myocytes. Consistent with this hypothesis, these investigators observed that the EHMT1/2 inhibitor UNC0638 restored the ability of 10T1/2 cells expressing IDH2-R172K to form fused myotubes. Similarly, primary RPT cells with an L2HGDH KD can overcome the block in tubulogenesis in the presence of UNC0638 (lowering levels of H3K9me3), although the cultures can also overcome the block in tubulogenesis in the presence of GSK343 (Taub, unpublished).

Shelar et al. [11] presented evidence that increased levels of methylated histones as well as DNA in ccRCCs with elevated L-2HG contribute to tumorigenesis. However, Shelar et al. [11] also provided evidence that the increased levels histone H3K27me3 in ccRCCS with elevated L-2HG are responsible for altering the genetic program of these tumor cells, and, as a consequence their state of differentiation. Indeed, the studies of Taub et al. [43] indicate that increased L2HG establishes a block in RPT differentiation, with associated epigenetic changes. Thus, it is of importance to consider the development of new avenues of epigenetic therapy for ccRCCs.

7. Conclusion

Recent clinical trials of epigenetic-based therapies in RCCs have examined on the use of DNA Methyltransferase (DNMT) inhibitors such as decitabine and azacytidine [47]. DNA methylation of tumor suppressor genes in RCCs is thought to contribute tumorigenesis, and the hypermethylation of an EGF response element (recognized by Krueppel-like factor 5 (KLF5)) is associated with poor prognosis of RCC patients [47]. *In vitro* studies concerning the effects azacytidine with RCC cell lines have also shown promise [48], and combination therapies are in progress [47]. This adds to presently prescribed medications including VEGF inhibitors (e.g. sunitinib) mTOR inhibitors (e.g. everolimis), and HIF2α inhibitors (e.g. belzutifan) [49]. However metastatic ccRCC continues to carry a 5 year survival rate of 13% [49]. Thus, new treatment options are critical.

Epigenetic therapy is pertinent not only for ccRCCs with elevated L2HG, but also for ccRCCs with other genetic alterations (which may occur in addition to reduced L2HGH levels). Recent genome-wide sequencing studies have indicated that a number of epigenetic modifiers and chromatin remodelers are frequently altered in ccRCCs including PBRM1, SETD1, KDM5C, KDM6A, and BAP1. Notably, ccRCCs often have a 50 kb deletion on chromosome 3p where VHL, PBRM1, BAP1 and SETD2 are located, which has opened up the door to individualized epigenetic therapy. SETD1 in particular is an H3K36me3 histone methyltransferase that plays an important role in DNA repair and genomic stability [50]. While mutations in SETD1 result in reduced histone methylation, mutations in KDM5C and KDM6A often result in increased methylation of H3K4me3 and H3K27me3, respectively. The genes encoding for these 2 histone demethylases are located on the X chromosome, and thus, when altered, can a permit an escape from X-inactivation of tumor suppressor genes. Unlike patients with SETD mutations, RCC patients with KDM5C and KDM6A mutations would be expected to benefit from inhibitors of specific histone methyltransferases.

In addition to epigenetic therapies, therapies developed against cancer stem cells may also prove protective against ccRCCS with elevated L-2HG. Several theories have been proposed regarding the origin of cancer stem cells, including that, a) cancer stem cells arise from normal progenitor cells which become tumorigenic due to undefined mutation(s), and b) that cancer stem cells arise from normal somatic cells that acquire stem-like properties through similarly undefined genetic mutations [51]. Thus, the block in renal proximal differentiation caused by elevated L-2HG is a mechanism that potentially results in the development of renal cancer stem cells. Recently, Fendler et al. [52] isolated ccRCC cancer stem cells which depend upon signals sent through the Wingless-related integration site (WNT) and NOTCH networks, which direct the formation of RPTs during renal development. Further studies are needed to assess whether the WNT and NOTCH pathways are active in ccRCCs with elevated L2HG, and whether the targeting of such pathways can alleviate the differentiation block caused by increased L2HG in normal RPT cells.

Acknowledgements

The Optical Imaging and Analysis Facility, The School of Dental Medicine, University at Buffalo, and The Confocal Microscopy and Flow Cytometry Center of the Jacobs School of Medicine and Biomedical Sciences of The University at Buffalo were instrumental in acquiring the results descried in the article. The research was supported in part by RO1CA200653.

Author details

Mary Taub
Biochemistry Department, Jacobs School of Medicine and Biomedical Sciences, University at Buffalo, Buffalo, New York, USA

*Address all correspondence to: biochtau@buffalo.edu

References

[1] Cantor JR, Sabatini DM. Cancer cell metabolism: One hallmark, many faces. Cancer Discovery. 2012;**2**:881-898

[2] Qi X, Li Q, Che X, Wang Q, Wu G. The uniqueness of clear cell renal cell carcinoma: Summary of the process and abnormality of glucose metabolism and lipid metabolism in ccRCC. Frontiers in Oncology. 2021;**11**:727778

[3] Semenza GL. HIF-1 mediates the Warburg effect in clear cell renal carcinoma. Journal of Bioenergetics and Biomembranes. 2007;**39**:231-234

[4] Menendez JA, Alarcon T, Joven J. Gerometabolites: The pseudohypoxic aging side of cancer oncometabolites. Cell Cycle. 2014;**13**:699-709

[5] Xiao M, Yang H, Xu W, Ma S, Lin H, Zhu H, et al. Inhibition of alpha-KG-dependent histone and DNA demethylases by fumarate and succinate that are accumulated in mutations of FH and SDH tumor suppressors. Genes & Development. 2012;**26**:1326-1338

[6] Wang JH, Chen WL, Li JM, Wu SF, Chen TL, Zhu YM, et al. Prognostic significance of 2-hydroxyglutarate levels in acute myeloid leukemia in China. Proceedings of the National Academy of Sciences of the United States of America. 2013;**110**:17017-17022

[7] Struys EA. 2-Hydroxyglutarate is not a metabolite; D-2-hydroxyglutarate and L-2-hydroxyglutarate are! Proceedings of the National Academy of Sciences of the United States of America. 2013;**110**:E4939

[8] Kranendijk M, Struys EA, Salomons GS, Van der Knaap MS, Jakobs C. Progress in understanding 2-hydroxyglutaric acidurias. Journal of Inherited Metabolic Disease. 2012;**35**:571-587

[9] Intlekofer AM, Wang B, Liu H, Shah H, Carmona-Fontaine C, Rustenburg AS, et al. L-2-Hydroxyglutarate production arises from noncanonical enzyme function at acidic pH. Nature Chemical Biology. 2017;**13**:494-500

[10] Shim EH, Livi CB, Rakheja D, Tan J, Benson D, Parekh V, et al. L-2-Hydroxyglutarate: An epigenetic modifier and putative oncometabolite in renal cancer. Cancer Discovery. 2014;**4**:1290-1298

[11] Shelar S, Shim EH, Brinkley GJ, Kundu A, Carobbio F, Poston T, et al. Biochemical and epigenetic insights into L-2-Hydroxyglutarate, a potential therapeutic target in renal cancer. Clinical Cancer Research. 2018;**24**:6433-6446

[12] Intlekofer AM, Dematteo RG, Venneti S, Finley LW, Lu C, Judkins AR, et al. Hypoxia induces production of L-2-Hydroxyglutarate. Cell Metabolism. 2015;**22**:304-311

[13] Chowdhury R, Yeoh KK, Tian YM, Hillringhaus L, Bagg EA, Rose NR, et al. The oncometabolite 2-hydroxyglutarate inhibits histone lysine demethylases. EMBO Reports. 2011;**12**:463-469

[14] Johansson C, Tumber A, Che K, Cain P, Nowak R, Gileadi C, et al. The roles of Jumonji-type oxygenases in human disease. Epigenomics. 2014;**6**:89-120

[15] Husmann D, Gozani O. Histone lysine methyltransferases in biology and disease. Nature Structural & Molecular Biology. 2019;**26**:880-889

[16] Scourzic L, Mouly E, Bernard OA. TET proteins and the control of cytosine demethylation in cancer. Genome Medicine. 2015;7:9

[17] Ye D, Guan KL, Xiong Y. Metabolism, activity, and targeting of D- and L-2-Hydroxyglutarates. Trends Cancer. 2018;**4**:151-165

[18] Lu C, Ward PS, Kapoor GS, Rohle D, Turcan S, Abdel-Wahab O, et al. IDH mutation impairs histone demethylation and results in a block to cell differentiation. Nature. 2012;**483**:474-478

[19] Schvartzman JM, Reuter VP, Koche RP, Thompson CB. 2-hydroxyglutarate inhibits MyoD-mediated differentiation by preventing H3K9 demethylation. Proceedings of the National Academy of Sciences of the United States of America. 2019;**116**:12851-12856

[20] Lindgren D, Eriksson P, Krawczyk K, Nilsson H, Hansson J, Veerla S, et al. Cell-type-specific gene programs of the Normal human nephron define kidney cancer subtypes. Cell Reports. 2017;**20**:1476-1489

[21] Brunskill EW, Aronow BJ, Georgas K, Rumballe B, Valerius MT, Aronow J, et al. Atlas of gene expression in the developing kidney at microanatomic resolution. Developmental Cell. 2008;**15**:781-791

[22] Mukherjee M, DeRiso J, Janga M, Fogarty E, Surendran K. Foxi1 inactivation rescues loss of principal cell fate selection in Hes1-deficient kidneys but does not ensure maintenance of principal cell gene expression. Developmental Biology. 2020;**466**:1-11

[23] Guo X, Zhang Q. The emerging role of histone demethylases in renal cell carcinoma. Journal of Kidney Cancer VHL. 2017;**4**:1-5

[24] Kang W, Zhang M, Wang Q, Gu D, Huang Z, Wang H, et al. The SLC family are candidate diagnostic and prognostic biomarkers in clear cell renal cell carcinoma. BioMed Research International. 2020;**2020**:1932948

[25] Hurtado, Del Pozo C, Garreta E, Izpisua Belmonte JC, Montserrat N. Modeling epigenetic modifications in renal development and disease with organoids and genome editing. Disease Models & Mechanisms. 2018;**11**:1-17

[26] Ishihara H, Yamashita S, Liu YY, Hattori N, El-Omar O, Ikeda T, et al. Genetic and epigenetic profiling indicates the proximal tubule origin of renal cancers in end-stage renal disease. Cancer Science. 2020;**111**:4276-4287

[27] Harlander S, Schonenberger D, Toussaint NC, Prummer M, Catalano A, Brandt L, et al. Combined mutation in Vhl, Trp53 and Rb1 causes clear cell renal cell carcinoma in mice. Nature Medicine. 2017;**23**:869-877

[28] Dubois V, Staels B, Lefebvre P, Verzi MP, Eeckhoute J. Control of cell identity by the nuclear receptor HNF4 in organ pathophysiology. Cell. 2020;**9**:2185

[29] Kalisz M, Bernardo E, Beucher A, Maestro MA, Del Pozo N, Millan I, et al. HNF1A recruits KDM6A to activate differentiated acinar cell programs that suppress pancreatic cancer. The EMBO Journal. 2020;**39**:e102808

[30] Lemm I, Lingott A, Pogge E, Strandmann V, Zoidl C, Bulman MP, et al. Loss of HNF1alpha function in human renal cell carcinoma: Frequent mutations in the VHL gene but not the HNF1alpha gene. Molecular Carcinogenesis. 1999;**24**:305-314

[31] Zhang G, An X, Zhao H, Zhang Q, Zhao H. Long non-coding RNA HNF1A-AS1 promotes cell proliferation and invasion via regulating miR-17-5p in non-small cell lung cancer. Biomedicine & Pharmacotherapy. 2018;**98**:594-599

[32] Liu Z, Li H, Fan S, Lin H, Lian W. STAT3-induced upregulation of long noncoding RNA HNF1A-AS1 promotes the progression of oral squamous cell carcinoma via activating Notch signaling pathway. Cancer Biology & Therapy. 2019;**20**:444-453

[33] Taub M. Primary kidney proximal tubule cells. Methods in Molecular Biology. 2005;**290**:231-247

[34] Taub M, Axelson E, Park JH. Colloidal silica-coated tissue culture dishes for primary cell cultures: Growth of rabbit renal proximal tubule cells. BioTechniques. 1998;**25**:990-994

[35] Han HJ, Park SH, Koh HJ, Taub M. Mechanism of regulation of Na+ transport by angiotensin II in primary renal cells. Kidney International. 2000;**57**:2457-2467

[36] Taub M. Gene level regulation of Na,K-ATPase in the renal proximal tubule is controlled by two independent but interacting regulatory mechanisms involving salt inducible kinase 1 and CREB-regulated transcriptional coactivators. International Journal of Molecular Sciences. 2018;**19**:2086-2095

[37] Berquin IM, Min Y, Wu R, Wu J, Perry D, Cline JM, et al. Modulation of prostate cancer genetic risk by omega-3 and omega-6 fatty acids. The Journal of Clinical Investigation. 2007;**117**:1866-1875

[38] Kleinman HK, Martin GR. Matrigel: Basement membrane matrix with biological activity. Seminars in Cancer Biology. 2005;**15**:378-386

[39] Taub M, Wang Y, Szczesny TM, Kleinman HK. Epidermal growth factor or transforming growth factor alpha is required for kidney tubulogenesis in matrigel cultures in serum-free medium. Proceedings of the National Academy of Sciences of the United States of America. 1990;**87**:4002-4006

[40] Chung SD, Alavi N, Livingston D, Hiller S, Taub M. Characterization of primary rabbit kidney cultures that express proximal tubule functions in a hormonally defined medium. The Journal of Cell Biology. 1982;**95**:118-126

[41] Han HJ, Sigurdson WJ, Nickerson PA, Taub M. Both mitogen activated protein kinase and the mammalian target of rapamycin modulate the development of functional renal proximal tubules in matrigel. Journal of Cell Science. 2004;**117**:1821-1833

[42] Chan K, Li X. Current epigenetic insights in kidney development. Genes (Basel). 2021;**12**:1281

[43] Taub M, Mahmoudzadeh NH, Tennessen JM, Sudarshan S. Renal oncometabolite L-2-hydroxyglutarate imposes a block in kidney tubulogenesis: Evidence for an epigenetic basis for the L-2HG-induced impairment of differentiation. Front Endocrinol (Lausanne). 2022;**13**:932286

[44] Pelletier L, Rebouissou S, Vignjevic D, Bioulac-Sage P, Zucman-Rossi J. HNF1alpha inhibition triggers epithelial-mesenchymal transition in human liver cancer cell lines. BMC Cancer. 2011;**11**:427

[45] Xu W, Yang H, Liu Y, Yang Y, Wang P, Kim SH, et al. Oncometabolite 2-hydroxyglutarate is a competitive inhibitor of alpha-ketoglutarate-dependent dioxygenases. Cancer Cell. 2011;**19**:17-30

[46] Tateishi K, Wakimoto H, Iafrate AJ, Tanaka S, Loebel F, Lelic N, et al. Extreme vulnerability of IDH1 mutant cancers to NAD+ depletion. Cancer Cell. 2015;**28**:773-784

[47] Hong SH, Jang EB, Park SY, Moon H-S, Yoon YE. Epigenetic approaches to the treatment of renal cell cancer. Korean Journal of Urology and Oncology. 2020;**18**:78-90

[48] Ricketts CJ, Morris MR, Gentle D, Shuib S, Brown M, Clarke N, et al. Methylation profiling and evaluation of demethylating therapy in renal cell carcinoma. Clinical Epigenetics. 2013;**5**:16

[49] Serzan MT, Atkins MB. Current and emerging therapies for first line treatment of metastatic clear cell renal cell carcinoma. Journal of Cancer Metastasis Treatment. 2021;**7**:127-137

[50] Angulo JC, Manini C, Lopez JI, Pueyo A, Colas B, Ropero S. The role of epigenetics in the progression of clear cell renal cell carcinoma and the basis for future epigenetic treatments. Cancers (Basel). 2021;**13**:2071

[51] Yu Z, Pestell TG, Lisanti MP, Pestell RG. Cancer stem cells. The International Journal of Biochemistry & Cell Biology. 2012;**44**:2144-2151

[52] Fendler A, Bauer D, Busch J, Jung K, Wulf-Goldenberg A, Kunz S, et al. Inhibiting WNT and NOTCH in renal cancer stem cells and the implications for human patients. Nature Communications. 2020;**11**:929

Chapter 3

Clear Cell Renal Cancer, a Tumour with Neuroendocrine Features Originating from the Erythropoietin-Producing Cell

Helge Waldum and Patricia Mjønes

Abstract

The dominating type of kidney cancer is the clear cell renal cell cancer (ccRCC), hitherto been thought to develop from proximal tubule cells. However, the ability of tubule cells to proliferate is at best controversial. ccRCCs show many peculiarities like erythrocytosis due to erythropoietin overproduction and a combination of early metastases and sometimes apparent dormancy and late recurrence, features in common with neuroendocrine tumours (NETs). We have shown that most ccRCCs express erythropoietin and the neuroendocrine marker neuron-specific enolase, and other neuroendocrine markers in a percentage of the cancers. Missense mutation in von Hippel–Lindau (VHL) factor is rather specific for ccRCC found in familial and sporadic forms. The function of VHL factor is together with other proteins to destroy hypoxia-inducible factors (HIFs), central in adaptation to hypoxia. Lack of functioning VHL factor results in continuous overstimulation of the erythropoietin-producing cell to release erythropoietin and parallelly to proliferate, and in long-term mutations and malignant transformation. Thus, ccRCC occurs about 30 years later in sporadic cases compared with familial von Hippel–Lindau syndrome, reflecting the time necessary for two versus one genetic change. Embryologically, there are many arguments favouring neural crest origin of the erythropoietin-producing cell.

Keywords: classification of kidney cancer, clear cell renal cell cancer, erythropoietin, erythropoietin-producing cell, neural crest, von Hippel–Lindau syndrome

1. Introduction

The kidney is not among the most common locations for cancer development, but kidney cancers often affect middle-aged people, and the mortality is high. Clear cell renal cancer cell (ccRCC) (also called conventional RCC (cRCC)) makes up about 80% of renal malignancies [1] and is accordingly the most important renal cancer. ccRCC may be accompanied by erythrocytosis which has been presumed to be due to production of erythropoietin (EPO) by the erythropoietin-producing cell (EPC) localised in the kidney. Some years ago, we showed that virtually all ccRCC cancer tumour cells expressed erythropoietin as well as the neuroendocrine marker neuron-specific enolase [2], which may suggest that the cell of origin of ccRCC is the EPC [3]. The present review is a follow-up further discussing the cell of origin of ccRCC.

2. Kidney cancers

Kidney cancers are classified according to presumed cell of origin with renal cell carcinomas making up about 90% [4]. Renal cell cancers consist of subgroups based on histological classification into ccRCC, papillary and chromophobe subgroups. ccRCC and papillary renal cell cancers (pRCCs) have been presumed to originate from proximal tubular cells. However, most cells in the adult kidney do not have the ability to divide and thus replace damaged or dead specialised cells [5]. Therefore, replacement of damaged nephrons does not occur after birth [6]. Generally, it may be noted that it seems strange that nephron cells with absent or at best low reproductive capacity should be the main origin of tumours. Based on gene expressions with similarities between proximal tubular cells and ccRCCs [7, 8], tubular cells have been thought to develop into ccRCC. However, discrepant expressions between normal proximal tubule cells and tumours presumed to originate from proximal tubule cells like ccRCC and pRCCs have been described [9]. In a review in 2012, it was written that the cells of origin RCCs "are far from established and only inferred by accumulated weight of marker similarities" [10]. Similarly, the degree of tubule regeneration and which cell type contributing to this process were discussed in a review in 2016 [11]. Recently, a novel stem cell subtype analysis for ccRCC based on stem cell markers was reported, but apparently not compared to any mature cells of the nephron [12]. It may, therefore, be concluded that there are uncertainties regarding the cell of origin of ccRCCs. Considering the classification of kidney tumours in general, the continuous changes and additions of new types [13, 14] indicate a weakness in the system and may suggest that the classifications are not rooted in biology. Our finding of erythropoietin and neuron-specific enolase expression in virtually all ccRCCs may indicate that the EPC is the cell of origin of ccRCC [2, 3].

3. Erythropoietin (EPO) and the erythropoietin-producing cell (EPC)

In the late part of nineteenth century, French scientists described the association between atmospheric pressure and the concentration of red blood cells [15]. Thus, the concentration of red blood cells increased in members of an expedition to the Andes mountains [16]. A factor in serum was suspected to mediate this effect, and this was shown to be true when serum from anaemic rabbits had erythropoietic activity in normal rabbits [17]. Finnish authors named the postulated substance erythropoietin [18], and the dominating role of the kidneys in the production of EPO was shown by reduced stimulation of erythropoiesis in nephrectomised animals [19]. However, some EPO production also occurs in the liver [15]. Subsequently, EPO was identified as a glycohormone [20]. It stimulates erythropoiesis by interaction with a receptor (REPO) localised on progenitor cells in the red cell line like erythroblasts. The EPC in the kidney was long disputed. However, it seems now that peritubular interstitial cells are established as the EPC [21]. Interestingly, these cells had a neuron-like morphology and expressed neuron genes [21]. In the liver, EPO production was also found in

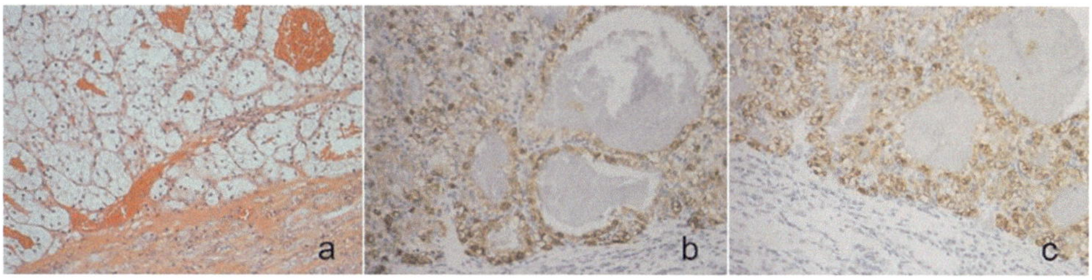

Figure 1.
Clear cell renal cell carcinoma examined by haematoxylin and eosin (a), by immunohistochemistry for erythropoietin (b) and neuron-specific enolase (NSE)(c). From (2) APMIS 2017; 125: 213–222. The figure is reused under the terms of the creative commons public domains declaration and with permission from the publisher.

cells surrounding the central vein in the liver [21], possibly stellate cells which have been shown to express EPO [22]. EPO has also been described in the brain [23].

The main stimulatory mechanism for EPO production and release is by the hypoxia-inducible factors (HIFs). There exist three O2 sensing HIF-α types (HIF-1α, HIF2α, and HIF-3α). HIF-1α and also HIF-2α affect many other processes than stimulation of EPO release including angiogenesis and other functions related to adaptation to hypoxia [15, 24]. HIF-2 seems to be the main regulator of EPO [25]. HIF-1α is ubiquitously expressed, while HIF-2α was initially reported in endothelial cells but has later been shown to be expressed in many other cell types [26].

EPO production in renal cancers, then named hypernephromas [27], was suspected based on erythrocytosis in some of the patients. A case report in 1977 described EPO production in a patient with ccRCC based on a biological mouse assay [28], and there is a report describing EPO production in a cell culture from a renal cell carcinoma [29]. EPO gene expression in ccRCC was reported to be much more common than the occurrence of erythrocytosis [30]. There are also studies evaluating the prognostic significance of EPO expression in renal cell cancers where one study did not find any effect [31], and the other reported reduced survival [32]. We cannot find that anybody had reflected on the EPC as the cell of origin in ccRCC before our paper in 2017 [2], where we found that most ccRCC expressed EPO in contrast to the other renal cell carcinomas which all were negative (**Figure 1**).

Before discussing cell of origin further, we will focus on clinical aspects of ccRCC, which also give strong indications of the central role of EPC in ccRCC carcinogenesis.

4. Clinical aspects of ccRCC

In the past, the classic symptom triad of RCC was haematuria, pain in the kidney area and a palpable tumour. However, nearly half of the patients do not have any symptoms suggesting renal illness [33], and in about half of the cases renal cancers are detected by ultrasonography or other imaging modalities done due to vague symptoms. Paraneoplastic syndromes are also an initial gateway to correct diagnosis. Among these syndromes, hypercalcemia, hypertension, polycythaemia, and Stauffer's syndrome (non-metastatic hepatic dysfunction [34]) are the most prevalent [35]. Hypercalcemia is due to parathyroid-related hormone (PTHrP), polycythaemia due to EPO, hypertension possibly due to renin, whereas the mechanism for Stauffer's syndrome is unknown. PTHrP elevation has been attributed to vascular endothelial growth factor (VEGF) expression in ccRCC [36].

Elevated erythrocyte sedimentation rate has for long been recognised to be a feature of renal cancer, formerly called hypernephroma, now ccRCC. Rising erythrocyte sedimentation may be an early marker for renal cell cancer [37] and also an independent prognostic factor [38]. C-reactive protein is also a predictive factor for metastasis in patients after potentially curative surgery [39].

Macroscopically, ccRCCs often are yellowish and small tumours often with an apparent capsule. ccRCCs metastasize at an early stage, and metastases are often present at diagnosis [40]. RCCs may metastasize to uncommon places as a finger [41], the pituitary gland [42], and skeletal muscle [43]. Moreover, first metastasis may manifest itself many years after apparent curative surgery as shown in a case report where a brain metastasis developed 15 years after surgery [44]. Late metastasis has been explained by early dissemination and tumour cell dormancy [45, 46]. Another possibility may be that the cell of origin due to inherent qualities like low expression of factors contributing to cell adhesion may cause metastasis spread at an early phase of malignant development when the proliferation still is rather low. Such a phenomenon may explain the so-called dormancy [47]. As we see it, the possibility that some cancer cells go to sleep and awake after many years does not seem very plausible, although until now it has been the prevailing theory [45]. Production of substances affecting the vascular bed-like dilatation reducing blood flow rate as well as increasing the vascular permeability could also be involved. We have previously described that the enterochromaffin-like (ECL) cell in the oxyntic mucosa of the stomach lacks E-cadherin [48] and also releases histamine which has profound effect on the vasculature [49]. The ECL cell has a very slow proliferation, which made some conclude that this cell did not have the ability to divide [50] which is not correct [51]. There may be an apparent mismatch between the fact that tumours prone to early metastasis are among those with tendency to occurrence of late metastasis many years after other manifestations of malignancy. This is typically found in tumours developed from cells with the capacity to metastasize at an early phase of the malignant process when the proliferation is still slow. Neuroendocrine tumours (NETs) [52–55] and melanomas [56, 57] developed from melanocytes which also are of neural crest origin [58] like the ccRCCs (see later) are among the cancers where late metastasis occur [44]. The dormancy accordingly most probably reflects tumours originating from cells with low proliferation but the ability to metastasize after only minor genetic changes.

Another peculiarity with ccRCCs is the anecdotal spontaneous regression of metastases after surgical removal of the primary tumour, a phenomenon perhaps related to the abscopal phenomenon (regress of tumour metastases outside the area of irradiation of other metastases) [59, 60].

5. Aetiology/pathogenesis

ccRCC is the dominating kidney cancer and is also the most aggressive form. The incidence of ccRCC is nearly the double in men compared with women [4, 61]. An explanation of this sex difference in occurrence is not known. Otherwise, cigarette smoking, obesity, and hypertension have been all associated with a slight increased risk of ccRCC [62], but the exact mechanisms have not been clarified. In Japan, heavy smoking was found to increase the risk [63], but the mechanism for the slight carcinogenic effect on the kidneys have not been clarified. In inhalation studies on rats, we examined the effect of nicotine added to the air in concentrations giving nicotine in blood exceeding that found in heavy smokers during greater part of 24 h for 24 months [64], or CO in a concentration giving about 15% carboxy-haemoglobin for most of 24 h for 18 months [65]. Although none of these studies were primarily done to explore possible mechanisms for tobacco smoking kidney carcinogenesis, the kidneys were examined macroscopically in both studies without finding any tumours. Thus, the mechanism for the effect of tobacco smoking on renal carcinogenesis is still unknown.

Obesity is an accepted and established role as a risk factor for ccRCC [62], but it is also associated with other types of cancers in other organs [66]. There exists a so-called obesity paradox between ccRCC and obesity, since obesity increases the occurrence and at the same time seems to improve the prognosis of the cancer [67]. Anyhow, a plausible mechanism for the carcinogenic effect of obesity is still not found. Likewise, on the background of the important role by the kidneys in regulation of blood pressure, it is not surprising that hypertension may be elevated in ccRCCs. However, again the mechanism for such a connection is not yet elucidated, although a role of the renin-angiotensin system has been examined.

On the other hand, a central role of the von Hippel–Lindau (VHL) tumour suppressor in pathogenesis of ccRCC is well established causing virtually all familial ccRCCs [68], but also the sporadic ones [69]. The average age at diagnosis of ccRCC as part of VHL syndrome is 37 years compared with 61 years of the sporadic form [40, 70]. Inactivation of VHL gene is only found in ccRCC of kidney cancers [40], and loss of functioning of both alleles of VHL gene may be common to all ccRCCs [40, 71]. VHL gene product (pVHL) binds to elongins making a complex which binds to the hypoxic-inducible factors, HIF-1 and HIF-2, which targets them to ubiquitin-mediated proteolysis [72]. Pathological elongins can also be a factor contributing to lack of proteolysis of HIFs. HIFs are released during hypoxia, and HIF-2 is being the main stimulator of erythropoietin release [25]. Our experience is that it is a close correlation between regulation of function and growth [73], which in this case will indicate that HIF-2 will not only stimulate erythropoietin release but also proliferation of EPC. Lack of proteolysis of HIFs will accordingly lead to chronic overstimulation of proliferation explaining the carcinogenic effect.

6. Neural crest origin of erythropoietin-producing cell

Most ccRCCs express erythropoietin as well as neuron-specific enolase [2]. Based on our study, it seems that both clinically (overproduction of EPO in a proportion of the patients), the central and universal role of HIF in the carcinogenesis of familial as well as sporadic ccRCCs and the universal and specific expression of EPO in most ccRCCs, these tumours are of EPC origin. A case report from 1989 also describes EPC expressing cell as the cell of origin of a ccRCC [74]. Moreover, clinically ccRCCs have as outlined above, many similarities to neuroendocrine tumours in general. Furthermore, polycythaemia due to EPO production has been reported together with somatostatinoma, paraganglioma, and phaeochromocytoma [75, 76]. We found not only EPO but also NSE expression in virtually all ccRCCs, but both markers, were mostly negative in the other types of renal cell carcinomas [2]. NSE has had a poor reputation concerning specificity, but when we did a separate study on NSE specificity comparing NSE with many other neuroendocrine markers and applying histochemistry with the highest sensitivity available, we found that NSE was expressed in all tumours which expressed another neuroendocrine marker [77]. Thus, NSE has unjustly been thought to be nonspecific due to its high sensitivity. Moreover, we detected synaptophysin expression in 6% and CD56, both neuroendocrine markers, in some ccRCCs [2]. It has to be underscored that during the process of malignant transformation, expression of markers from the cell of origin is gradually lost. Therefore, even expression in only a few percent of the tumour cells is of importance.

Interestingly, EPO production in neural and neural crest cells occurs in foetal life [78, 79]. In fact, EPO has been reported to play a role in the brain development [80]. Neural crest-derived cells have typically multipotential properties and play probably a very important role in carcinogenesis not only in the kidney but also for melanomas [81].

7. Conclusion

Evidence suggests that ccRCC is derived from the EPC, which upon hyperstimulation by HIF not only increases its EPO production but also is stimulated to proliferate. Genetic changes in VHL, either familial or sporadic, leading to loss of proteolysis result in increased concentrations of HIF. The EPC expresses markers compatible with neuroendocrine origin. A change in the nomenclature of ccRCC should be considered.

Conflict of interest

The authors declare no conflict of interest.

Author details

Helge Waldum[1]* and Patricia Mjønes[1,2]

1 Faculty of Medicine and Health Sciences, Department of Clinical and Molecular Medicine, Norwegian University of Science and Technology, Trondheim, Norway

2 Department of Pathology, St. Olav's Hospital – Trondheim University Hospital, Trondheim, Norway

*Address all correspondence to: helge.waldum@ntnu.no

References

[1] Mathers CD, Shibuya K, Boschi-Pinto C, Lopez AD, Murray CJ. Global and regional estimates of cancer mortality and incidence by site: I. application of regional cancer survival model to estimate cancer mortality distribution by site. BMC Cancer. 2002;**2**:36. DOI: 10.1186/1471-2407-2-36

[2] Mjones PG, Nordrum IS, Qvigstad G, Sordal O, Rian LL, Waldum HL. Expression of erythropoietin and neuroendocrine markers in clear cell renal cell carcinoma. APMIS: Acta pathologica, microbiologica, et immunologica. Scandinavica. 2017;**125**: 213-222. DOI: 10.1111/apm.12654

[3] Waldum H, Mjønes P. Time to classify Tumours of the stomach and the kidneys according to cell of origin. International Journal of Molecular Sciences. 2021;**22**:13386. DOI: 10.3390/ijms222413386

[4] Jemal A, Siegel R, Ward E, Hao Y, Xu J, Thun MJ. Cancer statistics, 2009. CA: a Cancer Journal for Clinicians. 2009;**59**:225-249. DOI: 10.3322/caac.20006

[5] Li H, Hohenstein P, Kuure S. Embryonic kidney development, stem cells and the origin of Wilms tumor. Genes (Basel). 2021;**12**:318. DOI: 10.3390/genes12020318

[6] Tögel F, Valerius MT, Freedman BS, Iatrino R, Grinstein M, Bonventre JV. Repair after nephron ablation reveals limitations of neonatal neonephrogenesis. JCI Insight. 2017;**2**: e88848. DOI: 10.1172/jci.insight.88848

[7] Lindgren D, Eriksson P, Krawczyk K, Nilsson H, Hansson J, Veerla S, et al. Cell-type-specific gene programs of the Normal human nephron define kidney cancer subtypes. Cell Reports. 2017;**20**: 1476-1489. DOI: 10.1016/j.celrep.2017.07.043

[8] Ishihara H, Yamashita S, Liu YY, Hattori N, El-Omar O, Ikeda T, et al. Genetic and epigenetic profiling indicates the proximal tubule origin of renal cancers in end-stage renal disease. Cancer Science. 2020;**111**:4276-4287. DOI: 10.1111/cas.14633

[9] Lee HW, Handlogten ME, Osis G, Clapp WL, Wakefield DN, Verlander JW, et al. Expression of sodium-dependent dicarboxylate transporter 1 (NaDC1/SLC13A2) in normal and neoplastic human kidney. American Journal of Physiology. Renal Physiology. 2017;**312**:F427-f435. DOI: 10.1152/ajprenal.00559.2016

[10] Axelson H, Johansson ME. Renal stem cells and their implications for kidney cancer. Seminars in Cancer Biology. 2013;**23**:56-61. DOI: 10.1016/j.semcancer.2012.06.005

[11] Lombardi D, Becherucci F, Romagnani P. How much can thc tubulc regenerate and who does it? An open question. Nephrology, Dialysis, Transplantation. 2016;**31**:1243-1250. DOI: 10.1093/ndt/gfv262

[12] Wang H, Xu H, Cheng Q, Liang C. Identification of a novel stem cell subtype for clear cell renal cell carcinoma based on stem cell gene profiling. Frontiers in Oncology. 2021;**11**: 758989. DOI: 10.3389/fonc.2021.758989

[13] Delahunt B, Srigley JR. The evolving classification of renal cell neoplasia. Seminars in Diagnostic Pathology. 2015; **32**:90-102. DOI: 10.1053/j.semdp.2015.02.002

[14] Cimadamore A, Cheng L, Scarpelli M, Massari F, Mollica V, Santoni M, et al. Towards a new WHO classification of renal cell tumor: What the clinician needs to know-a narrative review. Translational Andrology and Urology. 2021;**10**:1506-1520. DOI: 10.21037/tau-20-1150

[15] Haase VH. Regulation of erythropoiesis by hypoxia-inducible factors. Blood Reviews. 2013;**27**:41-53. DOI: 10.1016/j.blre.2012.12.003

[16] Viault F. Sur laugmentation considerable du nombre des globules rouges dans le sang chez les inhabitants dans des hauts plateaaux de l` Amérique du Sud. C R Academy Science Paris. 1890;**111**:917-918

[17] Krumdieck N, W.C. Erythropoietic substance in the serum of anemic animals. Proceedings of the Society for Experimental Biology and Medicine. 1943;**54**:14-17

[18] Bonsdorff E, J.E. A humoral mechanism in anoxici erythocytosis. Acta Physiologica Scandinavica. 1948;**16**: 150-170

[19] Peschle C, Sasso GF, Rappaport IA, Condorelli M. Erythropoietin production in nephrectomized rats: Possible role of the renal erythropoietic factor. The Journal of Laboratory and Clinical Medicine. 1972;**79**:950-959

[20] Miyake T, Kung CK, Goldwasser E. Purification of human erythropoietin. The Journal of Biological Chemistry. 1977;**252**:5558-5564

[21] Obara N, Suzuki N, Kim K, Nagasawa T, Imagawa S, Yamamoto M. Repression via the GATA box is essential for tissue-specific erythropoietin gene expression. Blood. 2008;**111**:5223-5232. DOI: 10.1182/blood-2007-10-115857

[22] Maxwell PH, Ferguson DJ, Osmond MK, Pugh CW, Heryet A, Doe BG, et al. Expression of a homologously recombined erythopoietin-SV40 T antigen fusion gene in mouse liver: Evidence for erythropoietin production by Ito cells. Blood. 1994;**84**:1823-1830

[23] Marti HH, Wenger RH, Rivas LA, Straumann U, Digicaylioglu M, Henn V, et al. Erythropoietin gene expression in human, monkey and murine brain. The European Journal of Neuroscience. 1996;**8**:666-676. DOI: 10.1111/j.1460-9568.1996.tb01252.x

[24] Lee JW, Bae SH, Jeong JW, Kim SH, Kim KW. Hypoxia-inducible factor (HIF-1)alpha: Its protein stability and biological functions. Experimental & Molecular Medicine. 2004;**36**:1-12. DOI: 10.1038/emm.2004.1

[25] Kapitsinou PP, Liu Q, Unger TL, Rha J, Davidoff O, Keith B, et al. Hepatic HIF-2 regulates erythropoietic responses to hypoxia in renal anemia. Blood. 2010; **116**:3039-3048. DOI: 10.1182/blood-2010-02-270322

[26] Wiesener MS, Jürgensen JS, Rosenberger C, Scholze CK, Hörstrup JH, Warnecke C, et al. Widespread hypoxia-inducible expression of HIF-2alpha in distinct cell populations of different organs. The FASEB Journal. 2003;**17**:271-273. DOI: 10.1096/fj.02-0445fje

[27] Kazal LA, Erslev AJ. Erythropoietin production in renal tumors. Annals of Clinical and Laboratory Science. 1975;**5**: 98-109

[28] Burk JR, Lertora JJ, Martinez IR Jr, Fisher JW. Renal cell carcinoma with erythrocytosis and elevated erythropoietic stimulatory activity. Southern Medical Journal. 1977;**70**:

955-958. DOI: 10.1097/00007611-197708000-00017

[29] Hagiwara M, Chen IL, Fisher JW. Erythropoietin production in long-term cultures of human renal carcinoma cells. The role of cell population density. Experimental Cell Research. 1984;**154**: 619-624. DOI: 10.1016/0014-4827(84) 90187-3

[30] Wiesener MS, Münchenhagen P, Gläser M, Sobottka BA, Knaup KX, Jozefowski K, et al. Erythropoietin gene expression in renal carcinoma is considerably more frequent than paraneoplastic polycythemia. International Journal of Cancer. 2007;**121**:2434-2442. DOI: 10.1002/ijc.22961

[31] Papworth K, Bergh A, Grankvist K, Ljungberg B, Rasmuson T. Expression of erythropoietin and its receptor in human renal cell carcinoma. Tumour biology: the journal of the International Society for Oncodevelopmental Biology and Medicine. 2009;**30**:86-92. DOI: 10.1159/000216844

[32] Michael A, Politi E, Havranek E, Corbishley C, Karapanagiotou L, Anderson C, et al. Prognostic significance of erythropoietin expression in human renal cell carcinoma. BJU International. 2007; **100**:291-294. DOI: 10.1111/j.1464-410X.2007.06978.x

[33] Gibbons RP, Monte JE, Correa RJ Jr, Mason JT. Manifestations of renal cell carcinoma. Urology. 1976;**8**:201-206. DOI: 10.1016/0090-4295(76)90366-6

[34] Tomadoni A, García C, Márquez M, Ayala JC, Prado F. Stauffer's syndrome with jaundice, a paraneoplastic manifestation of renal cell carcinoma: A case report. Archivos Españoles de Urología. 2010;**63**:154-156

[35] Padala SA, Barsouk A, Thandra KC, Saginala K, Mohammed A, Vakiti A, et al. Epidemiology of renal cell carcinoma. World Journal of Oncology. 2020;**11**:79-87. DOI: 10.14740/wjon1279

[36] Feng CC, Ding GX, Song NH, Li X, Wu Z, Jiang HW, et al. Paraneoplastic hormones: Parathyroid hormone-related protein (PTHrP) and erythropoietin (EPO) are related to vascular endothelial growth factor (VEGF) expression in clear cell renal cell carcinoma. Tumour biology: the journal of the International Society for Oncodevelopmental Biology and Medicine. 2013;**34**:3471-3476. DOI: 10.1007/s13277-013-0924-7

[37] Iversen OH, Røger M, Solberg HE, Wetteland P. Rising erythrocyte sedimentation rate during several years before diagnosis can be a predictive factor in 70% of renal cell carcinoma patients. The benefit of knowing subject-based reference values. Journal of Internal Medicine. 1996;**240**:133-141. DOI: 10.1046/j.1365-2796.1996.30195852000.x

[38] Choi Y, Park B, Kim K, Jeong BC, Seo SI, Jeon SS, et al. Erythrocyte sedimentation rate and anaemia are independent predictors of survival in patients with clear cell renal cell carcinoma. British Journal of Cancer. 2013;**108**:387-394. DOI: 10.1038/bjc.2012.565

[39] Johnson TV, Abbasi A, Owen-Smith A, Young A, Ogan K, Pattaras J, et al. Absolute preoperative C-reactive protein predicts metastasis and mortality in the first year following potentially curative nephrectomy for clear cell renal cell carcinoma. The Journal of Urology. 2010;**183**:480-485. DOI: 10.1016/j.juro.2009.10.014

[40] Cairns P. Renal cell carcinoma. Cancer Biomarkers. 2010;**9**:461-473. DOI: 10.3233/cbm-2011-0176

[41] Hopkins DT, Waters D, Manecksha RP, Lynch TH. Isolated soft tissue mass of the finger as the first presentation of oligometastatic renal cell carcinoma. BML Case Reports. 2022;**15**: e248718. DOI: 10.1136/bcr-2021-248718

[42] Öven BB, Demir MK, Çelik S, Moujawaz R, Somay A, Kılıc T. Isolated pituitary metastasis of renal cell carcinoma: A case report and systematic review of the literature. Current Medical Imaging. 2022. DOI: 10.2174/ 0929866529666220426121245

[43] Sun J, Zhang Z, Xiao Y, Li H, Ji Z, Lian P, et al. Skeletal muscle metastasis from renal cell carcinoma: A case series and literature review. Frontiers in Surgery. 2022;**9**:762540. DOI: 10.3389/ fsurg.2022.762540

[44] Choo YH, Seo Y, Choi J. Extremely delayed solitary cerebral metastasis in patient with T1N0M0 renal cell carcinoma after radical nephrectomy: Case report and literature review. Medicine (Baltimore). 2021;**100**:e25586. DOI: 10.1097/md.0000000000025586

[45] Friberg S, Nyström A. Cancer metastases: Early dissemination and late recurrences. Cancer Growth Metastasis. 2015;**8**:43-49. DOI: 10.4137/cgm.S31244

[46] Hadfield G. The dormant cancer cell. British Medical Journal. 1954;**2**:607-610. DOI: 10.1136/bmj.2.4888.607

[47] Waldum H, Mjønes PG. Correct identification of cell of origin may explain many aspects of cancer: The role of neuroendocrine cells as exemplified from the stomach. International Journal of Molecular Sciences. 2020;**21**:5751. DOI: 10.3390/ijms21165751

[48] Waldum HL, Ringnes E, Nordbo H, Sordal O, Nordrum IS, Hauso O. The normal neuroendocrine cells of the upper gastrointestinal tract lack E-cadherin. Scandinavian Journal of Gastroenterology. 2014;**49**:974-978. DOI: 10.3109/00365521.2014.909275

[49] Waldum HL, Hauso O, Fossmark R. The regulation of gastric acid secretion - clinical perspectives. Acta Physiologica (Oxford, England). 2014;**210**:239-256. DOI: 10.1111/apha.12208

[50] Barrett P, Hobbs RC, Coates PJ, Risdon RA, Wright NA, Hall PA. Endocrine cells of the human gastrointestinal tract have no proliferative capacity. The Histochemical Journal. 1995;**27**:482-486

[51] Waldum HL, Brenna E. Non-proliferative capacity of endocrine cells of the human gastro-intestinal tract. The Histochemical Journal. 1996;**28**:397-398. DOI: 10.1007/bf02331403

[52] Cunningham JL, Janson ET. The biological hallmarks of ileal carcinoids. European Journal of Clinical Investigation. 2011;**41**:1353-1360. DOI: 10.1111/j.1365-2362.2011.02537.x

[53] Tang M, Ai B, Ding L, Du J, Cheng G, Zhang Y. Late recurrence and metastasis of an appendiceal goblet cell carcinoid 24 years after appendectomy. Chinese Medical Journal. 2014;**127**: 591-592

[54] Dello Spedale Venti M, Giannetta E, Bosco D, Biffoni M, Carletti R, Chiappetta C, et al. Metastasis of lung carcinoid in the thyroid gland after 18 years: It is never too late. A case report and review of the literature. Pathologica. 2022;**114**:164-169. DOI: 10.32074/ 1591-951x-286

[55] Thai E, Gnetti L, Gilli A, Caruana P, Dalla Valle R, Buti S. Very late recurrence of an apparently benign pheochromocytoma. Journal of Cancer

Research and Therapeutics. 2015;**11**: 1036. DOI: 10.4103/0973-1482.154942

[56] Goodenough J, Cozon CL, Liew SH. An incidental finding of a nodal recurrence of cutaneous malignant melanoma after a 45-year disease-free period. BML Case Reports. 2014;**2014**. DOI: 10.1136/bcr-2014-204289

[57] Mansour D, Kejariwal D. It is never too late: Ultra-late recurrence of melanoma with distant metastases. BML Case Reports. 2012;**2012**. DOI: 10.1136/bcr.01.2012.5474

[58] Vandamme N, Berx G. From neural crest cells to melanocytes: Cellular plasticity during development and beyond. Cellular and Molecular Life Sciences. 2019;**76**:1919-1934. DOI: 10.1007/s00018-019-03049-w

[59] Shields LBE, Rezazadeh Kalebasty A. Spontaneous regression of delayed pulmonary and mediastinal metastases from clear cell renal cell carcinoma. Case Reports in Oncology. 2020;**13**:1285-1294. DOI: 10.1159/000509509

[60] Van de Walle M, Demol J, Staelens L, Rottey S. Abscopal effect in metastatic renal cell carcinoma. Acta Clinica Belgica. 2017;**72**:245-249. DOI: 10.1080/17843286.2016.1201614

[61] Bray F, Ferlay J, Soerjomataram I, Siegel RL, Torre LA, Jemal A. Global cancer statistics 2018: GLOBOCAN estimates of incidence and mortality worldwide for 36 cancers in 185 countries. CA: a Cancer Journal for Clinicians. 2018;**68**:394-424. DOI: 10.3322/caac.21492

[62] Dhôte R, Pellicer-Coeuret M, Thiounn N, Debré B, Vidal-Trecan G. Risk factors for adult renal cell carcinoma: A systematic review and implications for prevention. BJU International. 2000;**86**:20-27. DOI: 10.1046/j.1464-410x.2000.00708.x

[63] Minami T, Inoue M, Sawada N, Yamaji T, Iwasaki M, Tsugane S. Alcohol consumption, tobacco smoking, and subsequent risk of renal cell carcinoma: The JPHC study. Cancer Science. 2021; **112**:5068-5077. DOI: 10.1111/cas.15129

[64] Waldum HL, Nilsen OG, Nilsen T, Rørvik H, Syversen V, Sanvik AK, et al. Long-term effects of inhaled nicotine. Life Sciences. 1996;**58**:1339-1346. DOI: 10.1016/0024-3205(96)00100-2

[65] Sørhaug S, Steinshamn S, Nilsen OG, Waldum HL. Chronic inhalation of carbon monoxide: Effects on the respiratory and cardiovascular system at doses corresponding to tobacco smoking. Toxicology. 2006;**228**:280-290. DOI: 10.1016/j.tox.2006.09.008

[66] Vucenik I, Stains JP. Obesity and cancer risk: Evidence, mechanisms, and recommendations. Annals of the New York Academy of Sciences. 2012;**1271**: 37-43. DOI: 10.1111/j.1749-6632.2012.06750.x

[67] Hakimi AA, Furberg H, Zabor EC, Jacobsen A, Schultz N, Ciriello G, et al. An epidemiologic and genomic investigation into the obesity paradox in renal cell carcinoma. Journal of the National Cancer Institute. 2013;**105**: 1862-1870. DOI: 10.1093/jnci/djt310

[68] Latif F, Tory K, Gnarra J, Yao M, Duh FM, Orcutt ML, et al. Identification of the von Hippel-Lindau disease tumor suppressor gene. Science. 1993;**260**: 1317-1320. DOI: 10.1126/science.8493574

[69] Gnarra JR, Tory K, Weng Y, Schmidt L, Wei MH, Li H, et al. Mutations of the VHL tumour suppressor gene in renal carcinoma.

Nature Genetics. 1994;7:85-90. DOI: 10.1038/ng0594-85

[70] Pavlovich CP, Schmidt LS, Phillips JL. The genetic basis of renal cell carcinoma. The Urologic Clinics of North America. 2003;**30**:437-454, vii. DOI: 10.1016/s0094-0143(03)00023-5

[71] Dalgliesh GL, Furge K, Greenman C, Chen L, Bignell G, Butler A, et al. Systematic sequencing of renal carcinoma reveals inactivation of histone modifying genes. Nature. 2010;**463**: 360-363. DOI: 10.1038/nature08672

[72] Clifford SC, Astuti D, Hooper L, Maxwell PH, Ratcliffe PJ, Maher ER. The pVHL-associated SCF ubiquitin ligase complex: Molecular genetic analysis of elongin B and C, Rbx 1 and HIF-1alpha in renal cell carcinoma. Oncogene. 2001; **20**:5067-5074. DOI: 10.1038/sj.onc.1204602

[73] Waldum H, Mjønes P. Towards understanding of gastric cancer based upon physiological role of gastrin and ECL cells. Cancers (Basel). 2020;**12**:3477. DOI: 10.3390/cancers12113477

[74] Furukawa A, Kanda K, Yokozeki H, Maebayashi K, Kagawa S. A case of erythropoietin-producing renal cell carcinoma with a skin metastasis. Nihon Hinyokika Gakkai Zasshi. 1992;**83**:247-250. DOI: 10.5980/jpnjurol1989.83.247

[75] de Herder WW, Zandee WT, Hofland J. Somatostatinoma. In: chrousos G, de Herder WW, Dhatariya K, Dungan K, Hershman JM, Hofland, J, Kalra S, et al. Endotext. South Dartmouth (MA): MDText.com, Inc.; 2000

[76] Williams ST, Chatzikyriakou P, Carroll PV, McGowan BM, Velusamy A, White G, et al. SDHC phaeochromocytoma and paraganglioma: A UK-wide case series. Clinical Endocrinology. 2022;**96**:499-512. DOI: 10.1111/cen.14594

[77] Mjones P, Sagatun L, Nordrum IS, Waldum HL. Neuron-specific enolase as an Immunohistochemical marker is better than its reputation. The Journal of Histochemistry and Cytochemistry. 2017;**65**:687-703. DOI: 10.1369/0022155417733676

[78] Suzuki N, Hirano I, Pan X, Minegishi N, Yamamoto M. Erythropoietin production in neuroepithelial and neural crest cells during primitive erythropoiesis. Nature Communications. 2013;**4**:2902. DOI: 10.1038/ncomms3902

[79] Hirano I, Suzuki N. The neural crest as the first production site of the erythroid growth factor erythropoietin. Frontiers in Cell and Development Biology. 2019;7:105. DOI: 10.3389/fcell.2019.00105

[80] Yu X, Shacka JJ, Eells JB, Suarez-Quian C, Przygodzki RM, Beleslin-Cokic B, et al. Erythropoietin receptor signalling is required for normal brain development. Development. 2002;**129**: 505-516. DOI: 10.1242/dev.129.2.505

[81] Liu J, Rebecca VW, Kossenkov AV, Connelly T, Liu Q, Gutierrez A, et al. Neural crest-like stem cell transcriptome analysis identifies LPAR1 in melanoma progression and therapy resistance. Cancer Research. 2021;**81**:5230-5241. DOI: 10.1158/0008-5472.Can-20-1496

Section 2

Treatment of Renal Cell Carcinoma

Chapter 4

The Three-Dimensional Virtual Surgical Simulation and Surgical Assistance for Optimizing Robotic Partial Nephrectomy

Shuji Isotani

Abstract

Robot-assisted partial nephrectomy (RAPN) has been accepted as the standard treatment recommended for relatively small renal mass or even the T2 renal carcinoma in experienced hospitals as Nephron Sparing Surgery. To obtain better RAPN surgical outcomes, the understanding of surgical anatomies such as the position of intrarenal structure and the positional relationship of each structure should be detailed in a three-dimensional (3D) manner. The 3D virtual surgical simulation for partial nephrectomy based on the image segmentation method with high-resolution CT can provide the 3D anatomical details of the renal tumor focusing on their relationships with the arterial and venous branches as well as with the intrarenal portion of the urinary collecting system. This imaging application is also used as image guidance during the surgery, and it indicated that it provides the improvement of clinical outcomes such as the duration of hospitalization, transfusion, and major postoperative complications as well as conversion to radical nephrectomy or open partial nephrectomy. In this chapter, we describe the basics of the 3D imaging assistance methods for partial nephrectomy and the benefit of 3D virtual surgical simulation in optimizing the outcome of the RAPN.

Keywords: partial nephrectomy, robot-assisted partial nephrectomy, segmentation, 3D surgical simulation, image-guided surgery

1. Introduction

The number of stage 1 renal cell carcinoma has shown a significant increase in this decade. This trend was been brought by the improved modality of the screening imaging technology, such as ultrasound or CT imaging. The surgical treatment has been recognized as the standard surgical procedure for the treatment of early-stage renal cancer. Nephron sparing surgery (renal function-preserving surgery) has become the recommended treatment option for small-diameter renal tumors (small-diameter renal cancer) [1]. Comparing the oncological results after radical nephrectomy and partial nephrectomy, the outcomes of both surgical methods are equivalent; in addition, partial nephrectomy provides better preservation of renal function [2]. With partial nephrectomy, it may be considered lower the risk of cardiovascular and metabolic sequelae that would eventually turn into better overall survival for the patient comparing radical nephrectomy [3–5]. Therefore, at present, Nephron sparing surgery is positioned as the standard treatment for T1 small-diameter renal cancer. Partial nephrectomy is preferred for the following T1a tumors, and partial nephrectomy is recommended for T1b tumors between 4 and 7 cm, if possible [1, 6, 7]. Robot-assisted partial nephrectomy (RAPN), in particular, with the high-resolution 3D stereoscopic view and with multiple joints in robotic arms has been reported to have better treatment results than open surgery and laparoscopic surgery, such as preservation of function and reduction of perioperative complications [8, 9]. Today, at high-volume centers, the indication for partial nephrectomy has been gradually expanding with the robot-assisted procedure for selectedT2 cases. With increased tumor size and stage, PN becomes more challenging surgery, it may result in a higher risk of perioperative complications such as severe blood loss, urinomas, and arteriovenous fistulas. These are known as "Risk benefit trade-offs between partial and radical nephrectomy", so it was recommended that PN indication for large tumor should be considered more selective, and specific for patient and tumor factors [7, 10].

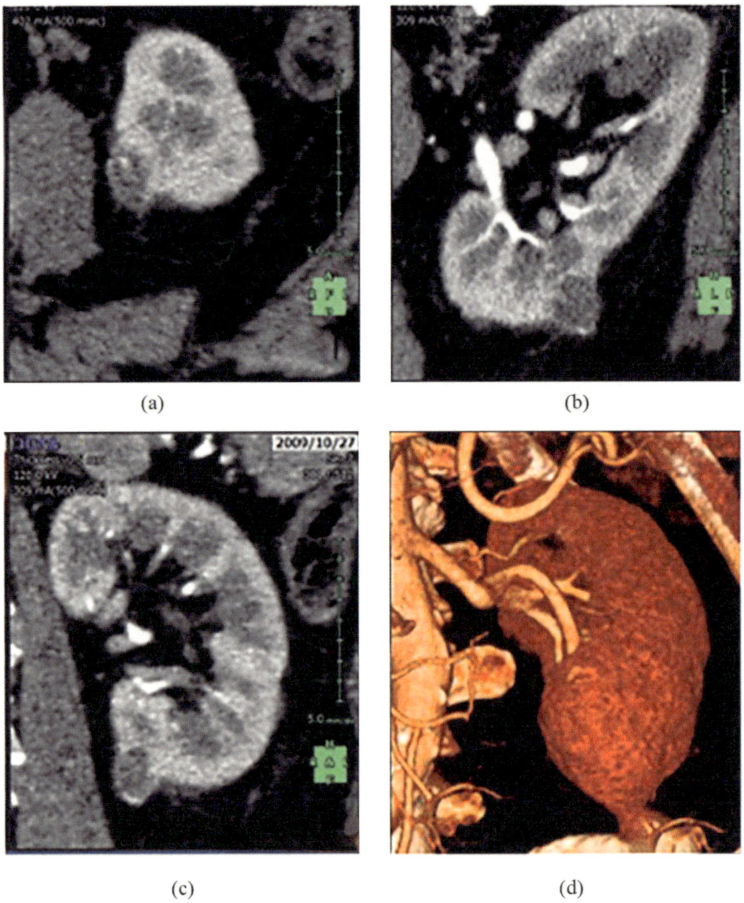

Figure 1.
The comparison of two-dimensional (2D) images of CT with axial (a), coronal (b), and sagittal (c) images and 3D CT volume rendering image (d).

Partial nephrectomy is a procedure that cuts into the blood-rich renal parenchyma, requiring complete excision of the tumor and precise repair of damaged renal structures. It was demonstrated that the degree of difficulty varies depending on the patient factors such as comorbidities or anatomical factors, and operators skillset and the learning curve is relatively long comparing other urological operations [9–12]. Due to the complexity of surgical procedure, it is considered that presurgical evaluation and surgical planning are quite important for each case. Surgeons should understand the surgical anatomy of the target kidney and tumor, especially, the position of renal structure, and the positional relationship of each structure should be known in order to optimize the surgical technique and achieve better surgical outcomes [10]. For a detailed understanding of the relationship of the hilum to the anatomy, it has previously been performed using two-dimensional (2D) image data (coronal, sagittal, and axial images) of computed tomography (CT) volume rendering for evaluation of these anatomical factors (**Figure 1a–c**) [13, 14]. Surgeons had to use their cognitive abilities to simulate the anatomy of the kidney and tumor as three-dimensional information while referring to those 2D images. For experienced urologists, it was probably easy to recall 3D information from 2D images; however, it is unclear whether all urologists can accurately reproduce the detailed anatomy and its complexity. Since 2012, there have been many reports to describe the befit of 3D CT volume rendering images for partial nephrectomy as the surgical support (**Figures 1d** and **2a**) [13].

However, only by the 3D-CT volume rendering, it was difficult to extract the urinary system or renal vein ant tumor at the same time, and it also enables to perform the volumetric analysis. To overcome the difficulties of 3D-CT volume rendering, one imaging technique called "segmentation" was developed as the image processing method (**Figure 2b**).

The segmentation process identifies the position information of each part of the organ and extracts one organ as a segment. Because the intrarenal anatomical structures of the kidney can be opaqued or removed as 3D models, interactive anatomical evaluation can be performed. It becomes possible to visualize the physical structure [15]. Since 2015, the Department of Urology, Juntendo University, has been using segmented

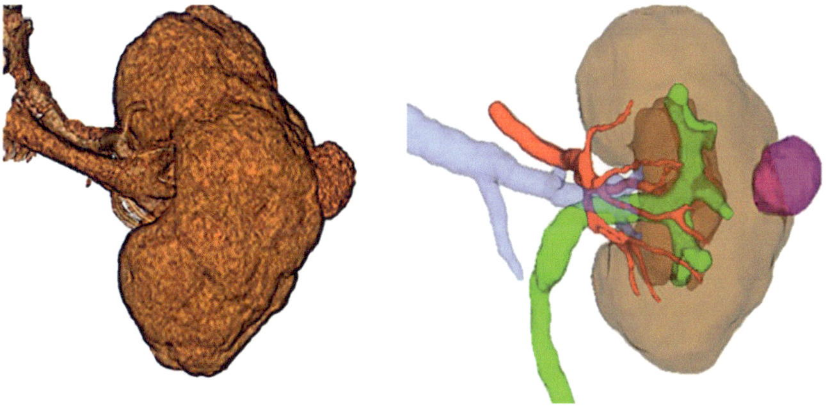

(a) (b)

Figure 2.
The comparison of 3D CT volume rendering image (a) and 3D segmented image (b). With 3D CT volume rendering image, it is difficult to distinguish renal organs at one glance. The 3D segmentation makes it easy to recognize the renal organs. This imaging process developed one step further to "image understanding" by recognizing organs as 3D images volume matrix.

3D images based on preoperative CT images to understand the anatomical complexity of renal tumors in RAPN and has been useful in preoperative planning [15, 16]. Furthermore, this imaging technology can also be used for surgical navigation during surgery and is extremely useful as an image reference during the actual surgery.

In this chapter, I will discuss the imaging technique for optimizing Robotic Partial Nephrectomy in surgical simulation and surgical assistance using 3D virtual surgical simulation.

2. Renal anatomical structures and 3D Segmentation

As mentioned earlier, at the partial nephrectomy, the surgeon cuts into the blood-rich renal parenchyma and removes the tumor and repairs damaged renal structures without hemorrhage and urine leakage. During all these processes, the surgeon needs to understand the detailed anatomy of the vasculature (renal artery and renal vein), urinary system, renal cyst, tumor(s), and other structures within or surrounding the kidney (**Figures 2b**, **3** and **4**).

In general, the renal artery is reaching from the main renal artery to the segmental artery, the interlobar artery, the arcuate artery, and the interlobular artery branch to the glomerulus. The anatomical distribution of renal arteries is divided into five segments including an apical, upper, middle, lower, and posterior segmental artery. Because each artery does not have adequate collateral circulation, the ligation of the segmental artery causes irreversible ischemia in that area of blood supplied by teach segmental filed [10, 13, 17].

This anatomical feature allows the surgeons to segmental resection only by segmental ischemia at the partial nephrectomy. All segmental branches arise from the anterior segmental artery, except for the posterior segmental branch, which arises from the posterior segmental artery. However, there are some anatomical variations are known in the distribution of the renal arteries. In the variation, the lower renal segmental artery may arise from the main renal artery. Also, there may an accessory artery also known as multiple renal artery or duplicate renal artery that arises from the

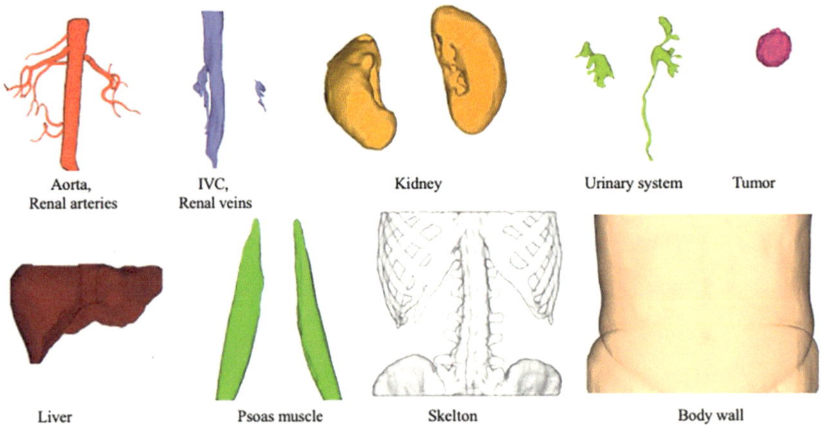

Figure 3.
At the segmentation process, renal anatomical structures the anatomical structures (aorta, renal artery, IVC, renal vein, kidney, urinary system, tumor, and other structures within or surrounding the kidney) are extracted from a different phase CT data using image recognition algorithm.

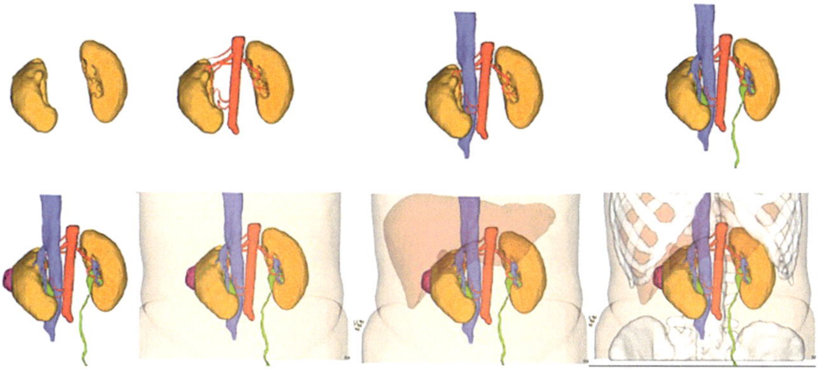

Figure 4.
3D structural images are combined together into one 3D image with registration technology. The extracted anatomical structures can change their transparency of the structural image for the easiest understanding, also organ volume such as tumor volume or renal volume can be calculated.

abdominal aorta directly and does not pass through the renal hilum [10]. The multiple renal arteries are regarded as the persistent embryonic lateral splanchnic arteries. The renal artery originally had multiple supply vessels from the aorta to the mesonephros during embryogenesis, but during the development process, two or more supply vessels remained on one side. The frequency of these duplicated renal arteries is estimated at 15% [10]. These anatomical variations of renal arteries have a great impact on actual partial nephrectomy surgery. If the surgeons know the detailed information about the anatomical distribution of the renal artery and operation time can be shortened and become safer and more reliable. The segmental clamping technique is one of the promising procedures to reduce the renal ischemic damaged area to preserve renal function. For effective segmental arterial clamping, the surgeon needs to identify the renal target artery in a 3D manner to get the essential ischemia damage for the resection of the tumor. Gill et al. reported super-selective arterial clamping in 2012 as the anatomical partial nephrectomy [18]. They used 3D segmentation to get the semitransparent tumor and renal arterial branches remain opaque. The 3D segmentation made it possible to see interrelationships of tumor vis-à-vis intrarenal segmental arterial branches, and such anatomical detail was necessary to operate on challenging tumors. The 3D segmentation is a medical image-aided tool that provides localization and assessment of organ size and shape. Kidney segmentation involves identifying the location information of each part of the kidney from high-definition CT, etc., and extracting one organ as a segment (**Figure 3**). The original computational 3D segmentation tool in developed in Japan in 2012 for the liver extraction tool and has been applied to the kidney in 2014 by Komai et al. [19]. In the past few years, 3D segmentation analysis for renal surgery has been applied in many countries, and it has been reported in some literature [19–24]. Today, with the computational algorithm, it is relatively easy to extract blood vessels from arterial phase CT imaging data. The renal arteries below 2 mm diameter and renal vessels are able to 3D segmentation by image recognition algorithm using the computer automatically. Also, the renal parenchymal and cortical regions can be extracted by the computational calculation with imaging software automatic tracing the edge of each kidney from CT images. The various image recognition algorithms were reported by researchers [19–24]. In addition, not only the blood vessels but also the renal tumor, the ureter, or the renal pelvis can be extracted automatically by using image recognition algorithms from the urography phase.

By combining extraction of the liver, bone, and body wall, now the surgeon can virtually reproduce all organ imaging required for performing the renal surgery by himself (**Figure 4**). The 3D segmentation processing improved medical imaging one step further to "image understanding," in other words "imaging diagnosis" by recognizing organs as 3D images volume matrix. By performing 3D segmentation processing, the 3D map of the kidney organs can be produced as the computational volume data. Since it is the computational volume data, it is possible to modify the visualization interactively and calculate the image volume easily. The anatomical structures can be seen by changing the transparency of the structural image, and each organ volume such as tumor volume or renal volume is calculated. In addition, image processing such as measuring and comparing the volume and cutting out the surroundings at a certain distance is possible.

3. 3D-virtual surgical simulation and 3D-image guided surgery

The idea of simulating surgery using medical images has been examined for a long time; however, it has rapidly progressed and spread in this decade.

The reason for this progress is the improvement in computational power used for image processing and the development of 3D image-processing software. They have become more powerful and cheaper than before, and they have come to be offered as affordable medical equipment. The 3D-virtual surgical simulation consists of the following four steps [1]. The first step is acquiring CT DICOM data and importing the imaging data to the image-processing software [2]. The second step is the

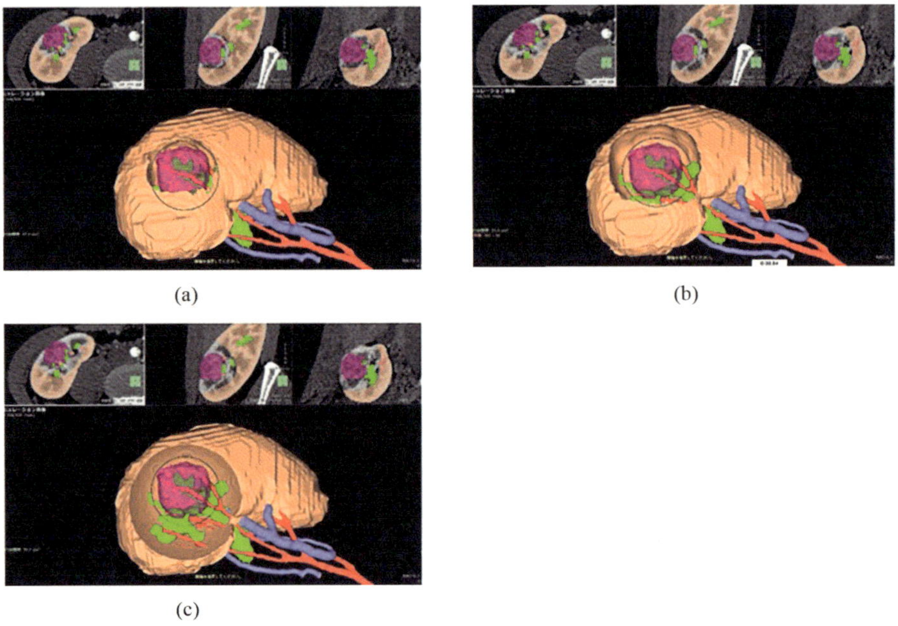

Figure 5.
In the surgical simulation, the surgeon can simulate the width of the resection margin size and resection method. Setting the cut surface with an optimal tumor margin with (a) resection margin; 1 mm, (b) resection margin; 5 mm, (c) resection margin; 10 mm. The surgeon can predict the involvement of the urinary collecting system or vascular system on the cutting surface by surgical simulation. The simulated resection volume and residual parenchymal volume can be calculated by CT volumetry.

segmentation of the renal structures (renal artery and renal vein, urinary system, renal cyst, tumor, and other structures within or surrounding the kidney) from a different phase of CT data, by imaging software (**Figures 3** and **4**) [3]. Then we perform 3D-virtual surgical simulation using the imaging software. With the software, we can simulate the two different resection methods, the enucleation technique and wedge resection technique, with any surgical margin size setting (**Figure 5**, Video 1). In the enucleation setting, the surgeon can simulate the width of the resection margin size for virtual enucleation. At the wedge resection setting, the surgeon can perform the simulation with setting by both the cut angle and resection margin for virtual resection. We can predict the involvement of the urinary collecting system with surgical simulation. If the urinary collecting system appeared on the planned cut surface, it means that the urinary collecting system was involved in the resection field, and the surgeon needs to decide to cut the collecting system or gently peel away it from the tumor. The imaging software also can calculate each resection volume based on CT volumetry and residual parenchymal volume of the healthy kidney [4].

The final step is the assessment of the arterial supply area for selective clamping. It is the computational approximation of vascular territories based on Voronoi decomposition. With this computational 3D Voronoi decomposition, renal arterial territories were calculated according to each arterial branch as the central point of the blood-supplied segment (**Figure 6**, Video 2).

For the 3D-image guided surgery, we connect the imaging software to the da Vinci system through digital video interface (DVI) input ports (**Figures 5** and **6**). We can see the real-time 3D-image surgical simulation on the surgeon's console of the da Vinci surgical system as the reference, using TilePro multi-input display. Initially, the surgeon's console display of the da Vinci shows the endoscopic view. In the use of TilePro, the images of 3D-image surgical simulation simultaneously appeared just

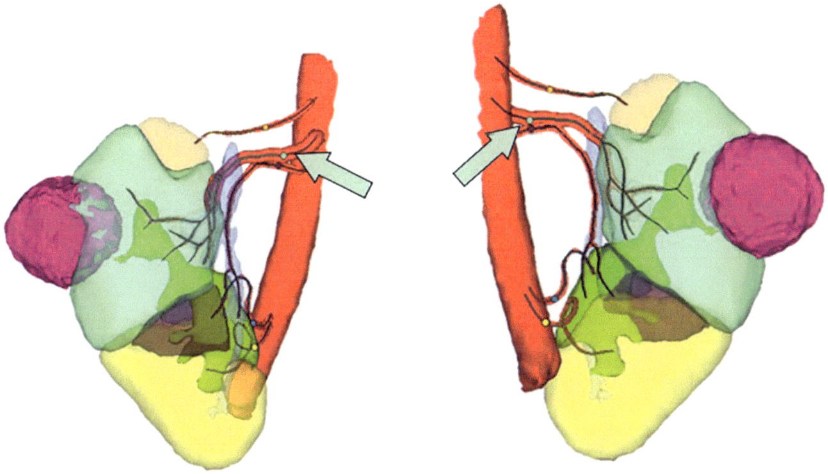

Figure 6.
The vascular territory (light green area) belonging to the selected targeted artery (light green arrow) branch is shown in a color-coded 3D model. The patient had five right renal arteries and a 2.5 cm tumor on the lateral side of the mid-renal pole. Vascular image analysis was performed to identify to know which artery supplied the tumor. Vascular analysis revealed that the second renal artery (light green arrow) is the only target artery to supply the tumor and 3 mm resection margin, so in this case, surgery was performed with a selective clamping technique on the targeted second artery only (the light green point was target point). The operation was safely completed without the need for an additional vascular clamp or blood loss.

below the standard endoscopic view (**Figures 7–9**), and the surgeon refers to their surgical plan to execute the same operation as they planned. The surgeon can identify the renal structures by manipulating the image in real-time 3D imaging; it allows the

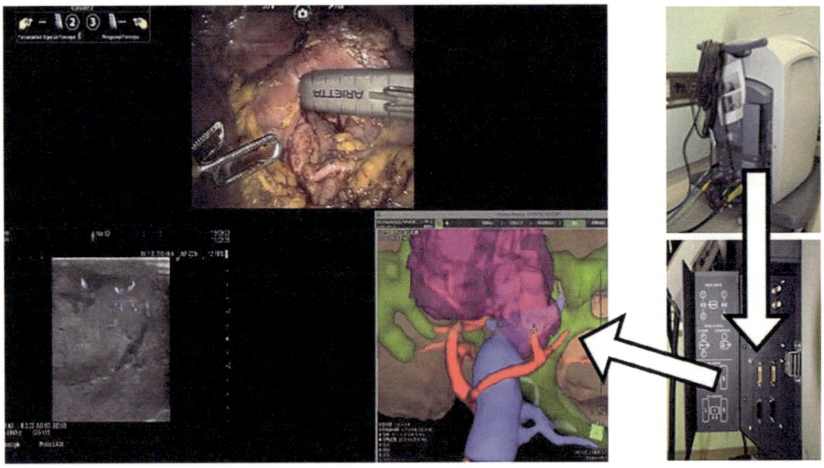

Figure 7.
The real-time 3D-virtual surgical simulation can be seen in the TilePro multi-input display on the surgeon's console of daVinci surgical system through digital video interface (DVI) ports on the backside. The simulated surgical plan in 3D volume-reconstructed images with key anatomical structures became available. The surgeon can identify the anatomical structure with ultrasound to complete the planned surgery correctly.

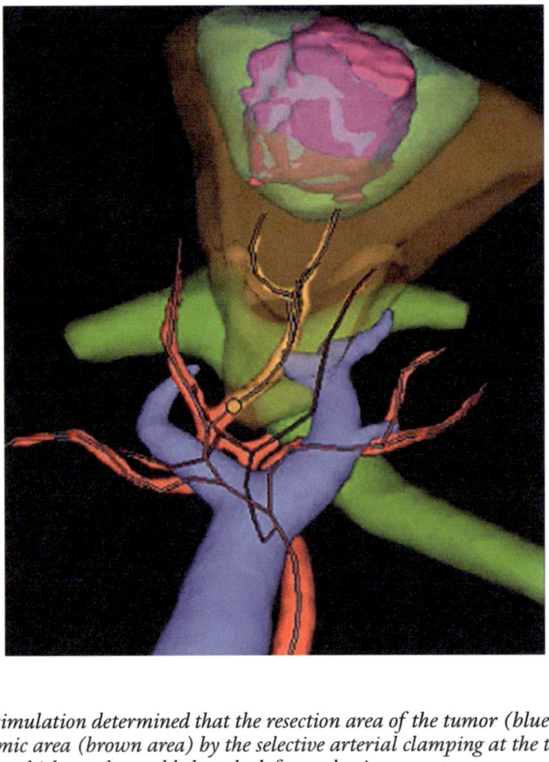

Figure 8.
The 3D-virtual surgical simulation determined that the resection area of the tumor (blue area), tumor (pink area), and regional ischemic area (brown area) by the selective arterial clamping at the third branch of the left renal artery (yellow dot), which was located below the left renal vein.

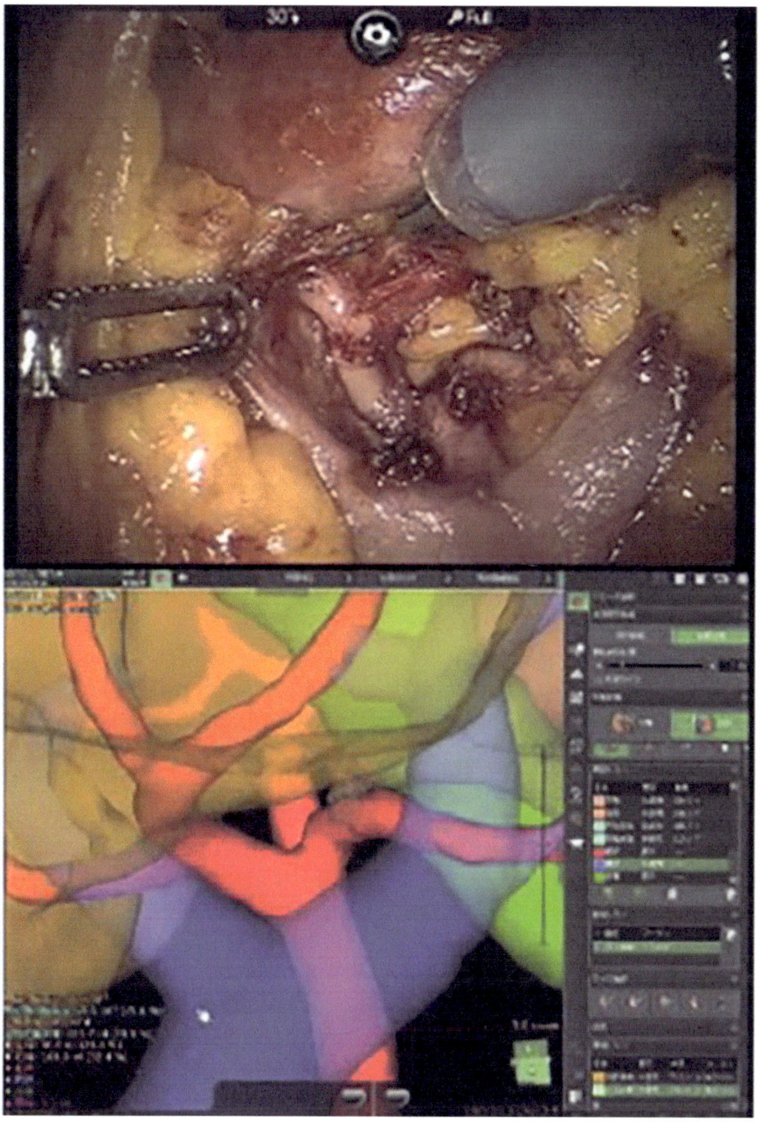

Figure 9.
A surgeon's console display with an endoscopic surgical view (top) and 3D-virtual surgical simulation (bottom) to identify the targeted vasculature after a renal hilum dissection. The top shows the actual surgical field, the renal arterial branches were already exposed at the second to third branch beyond the left renal vein. The bottom shows a real-time 3D-virtual surgical simulation image adjusted to the surgical field.

surgeon to find the key anatomical structures and cutting angle to adjust in the real operation field.

The Clinical benefit of the 3D-virtual surgical simulation and surgical assistance. Since 2014, there are some supportive publications reported about the 3D-virtual surgical simulation using this segmentation technology for RAPN from Japan. In 2014, Komai et al. demonstrated the surgical planning and surgical simulation by 3D segmented images for open partial nephrectomy [19]. In addition, in 2015, Isotani et al. reported that the 3D-virtual surgical simulation was able to provide the identification of tumor-specific renal arterial supply, prediction of collecting system opening, and prediction of postoperative renal function. They concluded that this imaging technique might suggest to the surgeons the best adjusted surgical margin size and arterial clamping point by virtual simulation [15]. Ueno et al. demonstrated that segmentation methods showed the prediction of urinary tract opening and the position of the opening as useful preoperative information [25]. Isotani et al. demonstrated in the video report in 2017, they showed the 3D-virtual surgical simulation and surgical assistance allowed for preserving renal function by minimizing the excision margin and limiting the ischemic area [16]. In 2016, Bernhard et al. reported their clinical experience with the 3D printing kidney models made from 3D-virtual surgical simulation with segmentation technology [26]. They demonstrated that this imaging technology also facilitate patients' pre-surgical understanding of their kidney tumor and surgery. As for the surgical outcomes, from Italy, there are some reports using the same segmentation technology. In 2018, Porpigli et al. showed that the 3D-virtual surgical simulation of the kidney with segmentation seems to promote selective ischemia to help in avoiding the global ischemia of the kidney compared to 2D CT [27]. In his report, he noted that in 90% of patients with 3D-virtual surgical simulation, the intraoperative management of the renal pedicle was performed as preoperatively planning, even though, in 39% of the group without 3D simulations group, the renal arterial pedicle management was intraoperatively changed [27].

In 2019, Porpigli et al. also showed that 3D-virtual surgical simulations were more precise than 2D standard imaging for evaluating the surgical complexity for partial nephrectomy. They showed a better perception of tumor depth and its relationships with intrarenal structures by 3D-virtual surgical simulation and resulted in predicting postoperative complications [28]. Additional supportive papers were reported by Bianchi et al. and Schiavina et al. in 2020 [22, 23]. However, even with the high-fidelity 3D simulation imaging, there was an absence of support for this imaging technology, which had a significant shortening effect on the total operation time or WIT (warm ischemic time) until 2021. Kobayashi et al. demonstrated in 2020 that the 3D surgical navigation system using the 3D-virtual surgical simulation showed preserving of renal parenchyma in robot-assisted partial nephrectomy, and it might contribute to improvement in postoperative renal function [29].

In 2021, Michiels et al. reported the significant benefit of 3D-virtual surgical simulation with segmentation in decreased warm ischemia time and reduced serious complications with the increased proportion of selective clamping. However, at the same time, they showed that the total operation time had been longer than without the 3D surgical simulation [20]. The longer operation time was due to the requirement of dissection of segmental arterial branches with risk of vascular injury. They concluded that the 3D-virtual surgical simulation and intraoperative guidance, the perioperative medical and surgical management may account for better clinical perioperative outcomes. These published articles supported that 3D-virtual surgical simulation may play an important role to refine patient counseling, surgical decision-making, and pre-and intraoperative planning for RAPN, and it helps to achieve precision surgical strategies and techniques according to the individual patient's anatomy.

4. Future development and options

Many articles suggested that by using 3D-virtual surgical simulation, the surgeon could have some benefit for Robotic partial nephrectomy. These surgical techniques, which combined with 3D-virtual surgical simulation and intra-op surgical navigation, may allow "Precision Surgery" to preserve renal function by minimizing the excision margin and limiting the ischemic area [16].

The future additional developments with 3D-virtual surgical simulation are the augmented reality (AR) in different surgical interventions [23] or registration of the 3D-virtual surgical simulation such as touch-based registration [19]. Even these some challenging articles have been reported, the accurate registration methods still have several problems or limitations to clinical usage [19]. No group has achieved that fully automated registration with noninvasive way during the current surgical RAPN workflow with quantitatively accessed registration accuracy. The future additional developments with 3D-virtual surgical Also, further areas may contain the automated segmentation method of the renal organs and incorporation of topological organ changes or tissue deformation by the human body status. Because it is known that the kidney has been moving up 10 mm cephalad and 11 mm medially in the flank position, and the respiratory motion makes the shifting the kidney in left-right, anterior-posterior, and cephalad-caudad directions.

These limitations suggested that ideally real-time registration methods to enhance the accuracy are required with endoscope data, updated with intraoperative ultrasound or touch-based registration [19].

5. Conclusion

Imaging surgery simulation in partial nephrectomy is useful for evaluating the difficulty of surgical procedures and for navigation during surgery planning and surgery, especially those using segmentation imaging technology. It is expected that such image processing technology will become more convenient and practical. In addition, image processing technology is expected to be incorporated and integrated into robot functions.

Additional video materials

Additional video materials referred to in this chapter can be downloaded at: https://bit.ly/3EDIo7Q.

Author details

Shuji Isotani
Department of Urology, Graduate School of Medicine, Juntendo University, Bunkyo, Tokyo, Japan

*Address all correspondence to: s-isotani@juntendo.ac.jp

References

[1] Ljungberg B, Albiges L, Abu-Ghanem Y, Bensalah K, Dabestani S, Montes SF-P, et al. European Association of Urology guidelines on renal cell carcinoma: The 2019 update. European urology. European association of. Urology. 2019;**75**(5):799-810

[2] Huang WC, Levey AS, Serio AM, Snyder M, Vickers AJ, Raj GV, et al. Chronic kidney disease after nephrectomy in patients with renal cortical tumours: A retrospective cohort study. The Lancet Oncology. 2006;**7**(9):735-740

[3] Go AS, Chertow GM, Fan D, McCulloch CE, Hsu C-Y. Chronic kidney disease and the risks of death, cardiovascular events, and hospitalization. The New England Journal of Medicine. 2004;**351**(13):1296-1305

[4] Kim SP, Thompson RH, Boorjian SA, Weight CJ, Han LC, Murad MH, et al. Comparative effectiveness for survival and renal function of partial and radical nephrectomy for localized renal tumors: A systematic review and meta-analysis. JURO. 2012;**188**(1):51-57

[5] Kaushik D, Kim SP, Childs MA, Lohse CM, Costello BA, Cheville JC, et al. Overall survival and development of stage IV chronic kidney disease in patients undergoing partial and radical nephrectomy for benign renal tumors. European urology. European association of. Urology. 2013;**64**(4):600-606

[6] Volpe A, Cadeddu JA, Cestari A, Gill IS, Jewett MAS, Joniau S, et al. Contemporary management of small renal masses. European Urology. 2011;**60**(3):501-515

[7] Mir MC, Derweesh I, Porpiglia F, Zargar H, Mottrie A, Autorino R. Partial nephrectomy versus radical nephrectomy for clinical T1b and T2 renal tumors: A systematic review and meta-analysis of comparative studies. European Urology. European Association of Urology. 2017;**71**(4):606-617

[8] Choi JE, You JH, Kim DK, Rha KH, Lee SH. Comparison of perioperative outcomes between robotic and laparoscopic partial nephrectomy: A systematic review and meta-analysis. European Urology. European Association of Urology. 2015;**67**(5):891-901

[9] Pierorazio PM, Patel HD, Feng T, Yohannan J, Hyams ES, Allaf ME. Robotic-assisted versus traditional laparoscopic partial nephrectomy: Comparison of outcomes and evaluation of learning curve. Urology. 2011;**78**(4):813-819

[10] Klatte T, Ficarra V, Gratzke C, Kaouk J, Kutikov A, Macchi V, et al. A literature review of renal surgical anatomy and surgical strategies for partial nephrectomy. European Urology. European Association of Urology. 2015;**68**(6):980-992

[11] Spana G, Haber G-P, Dulabon LM, Petros F, Rogers CG, Bhayani SB, et al. Complications after robotic partial nephrectomy at centers of excellence: Multi-institutional analysis of 450 cases. The Journal of Urology. 2011;**186**(2):417-421

[12] Kim SP, Campbell SC, Gill I, Lane BR, van Poppel H, Smaldone MC, et al. Collaborative review of risk benefit trade-offs between partial and radical nephrectomy in the Management of Anatomically Complex Renal Masses. European Urology. European Association of Urology. 2017;**72**(1):64-75

[13] Shao P, Tang L, Li P, Xu Y, Qin C, Cao Q, et al. Precise segmental renal artery clamping under the guidance of dual-source computed tomography angiography during laparoscopic partial nephrectomy. European Urology. 2012;**62**(6):1001-1008

[14] Shao P, Tang L, Li P, Xu Y, Qin C, Cao Q, et al. Application of a vasculature model and standardization of the renal hilar approach in laparoscopic partial nephrectomy for precise segmental artery clamping. European Urology. 2013;**63**(6):1072-1081

[15] Isotani S, Shimoyama H, Yokota I, China T, Hisasue S-I, Ide H, et al. Feasibility and accuracy of computational robot-assisted partial nephrectomy planning by virtual partial nephrectomy analysis. International Journal of Urology. 2015;**22**(5):439-446

[16] Isotani S, Stifelman M, Horie S. V3-04 precision surgery in robotic partial nephrectomy. The Journal of Urology. 2017;**197**(4):e289

[17] Ng CK, Gill IS, Patil MB, Hung AJ, Berger AK, de Castro Abreu AL, et al. Anatomic renal artery branch microdissection to facilitate zero-ischemia partial nephrectomy. European Urology. 2012;**61**(1):67-74

[18] Gill IS, Patil MB, de Castro Abreu AL, Ng C, Cai J, Berger A, et al. Zero ischemia anatomical partial nephrectomy: A novel approach. The Journal of Urology. 2012;**187**(3):807-815

[19] Komai Y, Sakai Y, Gotohda N, Kobayashi T, Kawakami S, Saito N. A novel 3-dimensional image analysis system for case-specific kidney anatomy and surgical simulation to facilitate Clampless partial nephrectomy. Urology. 2014;**83**(2):500-507

[20] Michiels C, Khene ZE, Prudhomme T, de Hauteclocque AB, Cornelis FH, Percot M, et al. 3D-Image guided robotic-assisted partial nephrectomy: A multi-institutional propensity score-matched analysis (UroCCR study 51). World Journal of Urology. 2021. DOI: 10.1007/s00345-021-03645-1

[21] Campi R. Case report: Optimizing pre- and intraoperative planning with Hyperaccuracy three-dimensional virtual models for a challenging case of robotic partial nephrectomy for two complex renal masses in a horseshoe kidney. Frontiers in Surgery. 2021;**8**:665328

[22] Bianchi L, Barbaresi U, Cercenelli L, Bortolani B, Gaudiano C, Chessa F, et al. The impact of 3D digital reconstruction on the surgical planning of partial nephrectomy: A case-control study. Still time for a novel surgical trend? Clinical Genitourinary Cancer. 2020;**18**(6):e669-e678

[23] Schiavina R, Bianchi L, Chessa F, Barbaresi U, Cercenelli L, Lodi S, et al. Augmented reality to guide selective clamping and tumor dissection during robot-assisted partial nephrectomy: A preliminary experience. Clinical Genitourinary Cancer. 2021;**19**(3):e149-e155

[24] Nimmagadda N, Ferguson JM, Kavoussi NL, Pitt B, Barth EJ, Granna J, et al. Patient-specific, touch-based registration during robotic, image-guided partial nephrectomy. World Journal of Urology. 2022;**40**(2):671-677

[25] Ueno D, Makiyama K, Yamanaka H, Ijiri T, Yokota H, Kubota Y. Prediction of open urinary tract in laparoscopic partial nephrectomy by virtual resection plane visualization. BMC Urology. 2014;**14**:47

[26] Bernhard J-C, Isotani S, Matsugasumi T, Duddalwar V, Hung AJ,

Suer E, et al. Personalized 3D printed model of kidney and tumor anatomy: A useful tool for patient education. World Journal of Urology. 2016;**34**(3):337-345

[27] Porpiglia F, Fiori C, Checcucci E, Amparore D, Bertolo R. Hyperaccuracy three-dimensional reconstruction is able to maximize the efficacy of selective clamping during robot- assisted partial nephrectomy for complex renal masses. European urology. European Association of Urology. 2018;**74**(5):651-660

[28] Porpiglia F, Amparore D, Checcucci E, Manfredi M, Stura I, Migliaretti G, et al. Three-dimensional virtual imaging of renal tumours: A new tool to improve the accuracy of nephrometry scores. BJU International. 2019;**124**(6):945-954

[29] Kobayashi S, Cho B, Mutaguchi J, Inokuchi J, Tatsugami K, Hashizume M, et al. Surgical navigation improves renal parenchyma volume preservation in robot-assisted partial nephrectomy: A propensity score matched comparative analysis. JURO. 2020;**204**(1):149-156

Chapter 5

Recent Advances and New Perspectives in Surgery of Renal Cell Carcinoma

Congcong Xu, Dekai Liu, Chengcheng Xing, Jiaqi Du, Gangfu Zheng, Nengfeng Yu, Dingya Zhou, Honghui Cheng, Kefan Yang, Qifeng Zhong and Yichun Zheng

Abstract

Renal cell carcinoma (RCC) is one of the most common types of cancer in the urogenital system. For localized renal cell carcinoma, nephron-sparing surgery (NSS) is becoming the optimal choice because of its advantage in preserving renal function. Traditionally, partial nephrectomy is performed with renal pedicle clamping to decrease blood loss. Furthermore, both renal pedicle clamping and the subsequent warm renal ischemia time affect renal function and increase the risk of postoperative renal failure. More recently, there has also been increasing interest in creating surgical methods to meet the requirements of nephron preservation and shorten the renal warm ischemia time including assisted or unassisted zero-ischemia surgery. As artificial intelligence increasingly integrates with surgery, the three-dimensional visualization technology of renal vasculature is applied in the NSS to guide surgeons. In addition, the renal carcinoma complexity scoring system is also constantly updated to guide clinicians in the selection of appropriate treatments for patients individually. In this article, we provide an overview of recent advances and new perspectives in NSS.

Keywords: renal cell carcinoma, zero ischemia, partial nephrectomy, tumor enucleation, renal carcinoma complexity scoring system

1. Introduction

With the development of screening techniques, increasing numbers of renal tumors are being diagnosed at an early stage without clinical symptoms [1]. Surgical resection remains the cornerstone of renal cell carcinoma (RCC) treatment [2]. Recent studies have shown that renal sparing techniques, such as partial nephrectomy (PN), achieve a comparable tumor prognosis and significantly improve perioperative morbidity and mortality. And guidelines from multiple urological associations recommend PN as the standard of care for early renal cell carcinoma [3, 4]. With the development of laparoscopic nephron-sparing surgery (NSS), urological surgeons strive to shorten the renal warm ischemia time (WIT) and preserve more renal parenchyma while removing tumor tissue. In order to preserve more renal parenchyma, laparoscopic renal tumor enucleation and renorrhaphy technique including deepsutures running the base of the defect, precise vesselsuture ligation, and no renorrhaphy at all have been developed [4]. In order to shorten the renal warm ischemia time, there are some surgical methods, such as microwave ablation/radio frequency ablation/laser/hydro-jet-assisted zero-ischemia laparoscopic partial nephrectomy (LPN), selective renal artery occlusion/embolization-assisted zero-ischemia laparoscopic partial nephrectomy, unassisted zero-ischemia laparoscopic partial nephrectomy and zero-ischemia laparoscopic renal tumor enucleation, and zero-ischemia laparoscopic partial nephrectomy by re-suturing [5]. Preoperative three-dimensional visualization technology of renal vasculature is increasingly used to implement multiple zero-ischemic approaches in laparoscopic nephron-sparing surgery [6].

The Mayo Clinic thrombus classification is widely used to describe levels of inferior vena cava tumor thrombus and is significant to guide the operation for renal cell carcinoma with venous thrombus in the open era [7]. But in the minimally invasive surgery era, Prof. Zhang et al. summarized a large number of surgical experiences of renal cell carcinoma with venous thrombus and put forward the "301 classification" system [8]. The system based on anatomical landmarks in which one grade corresponds to one surgical strategy improves surgical choice in the treatment of renal cell carcinoma with venous thrombus.

In this article, we summarize the various new surgical methods for renal cell carcinoma and describe the advantages and disadvantages of each of these methods. Moreover, we provide an overview of the latest research on RCC surgery and new scoring system which would help physicians to better personalize surgical treatment for patients.

2. Introduction of assisted zero-ischemia surgery

With increasing evidence indicates warm ischemia time (WIT) can have significant impact to minimize the loss of renal function after partial nephrectomy (PN), scientists are committed to reducing warm ischemia time, even achieving zero-ischemia surgery. Techniques trying to achieve zero ischemia are as follows.

2.1 Selective renal artery embolization technique

2.1.1 Methods

DSA superselective target artery embolization was performed in the interventional operating room 1 to 12 hours before surgery. Seldinger puncture method was used to insert F5 arterial catheter through the right femoral artery, and Yashiro catheter was used to perform renal artery angiography, superselected to the renal tumor supply artery, injected embolic agent, and then angiography was performed again to understand the embolization effect. Then laparoscopic partial nephrectomy with zero ischemia was performed [9].

2.1.2 Results

At 3-month and 1-year follow-up, the median increase of serum creatinine levels was 0.3 mg/dL and 0.24 mg/dL, respectively, and the median decrease of split renal function was 9% and 5%, respectively. The median tumor size was 4.2 cm (range, 2.5 to 6.5 cm). The median operative time was 62 minutes (35–220 minutes), the median blood loss was 150 ml (20–800 ml), and the median hospital stay was 3 days (2–12 days). None of the patients had end-stage CKD [10].

2.1.3 Complications

Complications are urinary tract infection, pulmonary infection, postoperative incision infection, postoperative intestinal obstruction, pelvic effusion and lower extremity venous thrombosis, as well as complications after superselective arterial embolization (low back pain, fever, infection, local hematoma), etc.

2.1.4 Advantages and limitations

With this technique, bleeding can be effectively stopped during surgery and the survival of the remnant kidney tissue can be maximized. The disadvantages of this technique are as follows. Firstly, superselective artery embolization is not successful in about 20% of cases, which is negatively correlated with the RENAL score. Especially in the face of large and endogenous tumors, the use of DSA to superselectively embolize the tumor to supply the artery needs more theoretical support [10]. Secondly, superselective arterial embolization can lead to edema and gangrene in the area of hand surgery, which brings difficulty to correctly distinguish normal tissue from tumor tissue. It is necessary to be vigilant all the time; otherwise, the tumor is easy to rupture and the positive rate of surgical margin will increase. For beginners, adequate surgical margin should be ensured from the tumor body. Thirdly, the use of iodine contrast and hemostatic agents could lead to contrast medium-induced nephropathy [11].

2.2 Selective renal artery occlusion technique

2.2.1 Methods

Nohara T and colleagues first introduced the concept of this technique in 2008 as a modified form of anatrophic partial nephrectomy [12]. First, the feeding branch of the tumor was determined by angiographic assessment or computed tomography angiography (CTA). During the operation, secondary or even tertiary renal arteries were isolated and vascular clips were used to control the renal segment arteries in the tumor area, and the renal segment arteries were isolated and blocked. The tumor and surrounding renal parenchyma were completely resected 0.5 to 1.0 cm from the tumor margin.

2.2.2 Results

Compared with total renal artery occlusion partial nephrectomy, the operation time and warm ischemia time were longer, and the intraoperative blood loss was more, and the differences were statistically significant ($P < 0.05$). One month after operation, the serum creatinine and urea nitrogen of the group undergoing superselective renal artery occlusion were lower than those of the group undergoing total renal artery occlusion, and the differences were statistically significant ($P < 0.05$) [11].

2.2.3 Complications

The injury of renal vein, renal pelvis, and ureter is a common complication when the renal artery is separated. As for postoperative complications, hematuria is usually caused by inadequate suture of renal pelvis and calyces during operation.

2.2.4 Advantages and limitations

It can not only provide a bloodless surgical field of view but also minimize the risk of ischemic injury and effectively protect renal function. Since only the branch of renal artery in the tumor area is blocked, the requirement of blocking time will be relaxed, which can allow more time for tumor resection and suture. However, compared with the main renal artery occlusion, the operation time is longer, the wound caused by vascular separation is larger, and the intraoperative bleeding is more [13].

2.3 Laser-assisted technique

2.3.1 Methods

The frontal laser fiber was used for vaporesection between 20 W and 25 W in all cases. The laser has the ability to coagulate and vaporize or cut, depending on the distance of the tip of the fiber from the tissue being resected (5 mm or 1–2 mm, respectively). After complete resection, the tumor was extracted through an endoscopic specimen bag via the 12- to 15-mm laparoscopic port [14].

2.3.2 Results

It is a good way to achieve minimally invasive surgery, helps to reduce bleeding in the case of complete tumor removal, and reduces the rate of positive margins [14].

2.3.3 Advantages and limitations

Carbon dioxide (CO_2) laser was the first laser used in clinical practice for partial nephrectomy. However, when neodymium-doped yttrium aluminum garnet (Nd:YAG) laser operated at 1064 nm (a 532-nm version exist for lithotripsy), it has a deeper length of tissue penetration (up to 1 cm) than CO_2 laser. Nd:YAG laser revealed promising results with excellent cutting and coagulation properties, but the deeper tissue penetration increased the risk of damage to healthy kidney tissue [11]. The newer thulium:yttrium-aluminum-garnet (Th:YAG) laser was first introduced into clinical practice in 2005. It has a wavelength of 2013 nm in continuous wave mode and could offer complete absorption of laser energy in water, providing superior vaporization and hemostatic properties than those of other lasers, which means the laser allows both excellent coagulation and vaporization/cutting capabilities [15].

However, laser coagulation and vaporization create a problematic smoke plume that can obscure direct operative vision during resection, as well as the laser does not have the ability to seal larger arterial vessels greater than 2.0 mm. Therefore, the potential for bleeding increases with deeper endophytic tumors [16].

2.3.4 Complications

Severe carbonization sometimes will be produced because of difficulty in control [16].

2.3.5 Advance

An ideal laser setup should provide accurate and adequate tissue cutting and ablation without causing carbonization, splattering, or excessive smoke. In that case, the operator could avoid the necessity for irrigation and vision would be improved during resection. In addition, in such an ideal setup, hemostasis should be completed safely even in larger blood vessels without suture or additional hemostatic agents. Finally, the ideal laser for the operator should be fast and easy to use [16].

2.4 Radio frequency ablation (RFA)-assisted technique

2.4.1 Methods

After opening the renal fascia, the renal artery was identified and suspended. Fat was removed from the tumor and surrounding tissue. The tumor location was determined by direct vision and laparoscopic ultrasonography. Before RFA, all tumors were biopsied using a 22-gauge TruCore®. To avoid additional puncture, the electrode was introduced through the abdominal wall or a laparoscopic trocar. Intraoperative ultrasonography was used to guide electrode insertion and monitor ablation, which could ensure thermal energy cover the tumor base. RFA was performed for 1 to 3 cycles for 6 to 12 minutes each depending on tumor size and depth [17].

2.4.2 Indications

The median tumor size was 3.2 cm (2.8–3.9), and the majority (73.1%, n = 133) were exophytic in more than 50% of cases [17].

2.4.3 Results

Xiaozhi Zhao reported that the glomerular filtration rate did not differ before versus 12 months after radio frequency ablation-assisted surgery, and 3-year cancer specific, cumulative, and progression-free survival was 100%, 97.3% and 96.4%, respectively [17].

2.4.4 Advantages

As the mass with a rim of normal parenchyma is coagulated with RF energy, minimal blood loss and good visualization were achieved during tumor excision. It can also prevent or delay the decline of renal function to the maximum extent [18].

2.4.5 Limitations/complications

When comes to disadvantages, the first is an increased risk of positive surgical margins due to the difficulty in identifying the tumor margin. For another, the placement of electrodes and the thermal penetration could be complicated by calyceal injury, urinary leakage, and venous injuries. In contrast, the incidence of urinary leakage seems to be higher than that of traditional nephron-sparing surgery (NSS) or tumor enucleation (TE) [18, 19].

2.5 Microwave ablation (MWA)-assisted technique

2.5.1 Methods

After the tumor was localized and dissected, 1 to 3 cycles of MWA were performed lasting 2 to 8 min depending on the tumor size and depth. Zero-ischemia NSS can be achieved using the MWA-TE technique by placement of the MWA electrode to create a relatively avascular plane [5, 20].

2.5.2 Indications and contraindications

For the patients with a single, sporadic, unilateral, organ-confirmed and pathologically diagnosed renal cell carcinoma were included in the study of microwave ablation-assisted technology [14]. And the patients with multiple tumors on ipsilateral kidney, collecting system or renal vein invasion, previous renal surgery history of the operative kidney, or with other renal diseases (such as renal calculi, glomerular nephritis, etc.) are not suitable [5].

2.5.3 Results

In a 3-year follow-up of 100 patients who underwent laparoscopic partial nephrectomy (LPN), Moinzadeh et al. reported overall survival (OS) of 86%, cancer-specific survival of 100% and recurrence-free survival (RFS) of 100%. A recent study of microwave ablation-assisted tumor enucleation for renal cell carcinoma shows no significant difference between preoperative, postoperative, and latest eGFR [21]. And the OS of 3- and 5-year was 99.6% and 98.4%, respectively, and RFS was 98.2% and 95.8%, respectively. Microwave ablation-assisted zero-ischemia laparoscopic technology is considered to be a viable and effective nephron-sparing surgical technique for selected renal tumors, with a low perioperative complication rate and promising mid-to-long-term oncological and functional outcomes [5].

2.5.4 Advantages

MWA causes coagulated cell necrosis by inducing friction of water molecules. Compared to RFA, MWA is more effective for the ablation of larger tumors due to its heat generation mechanism. In clinical practice, we found that MWA has the advantages of higher intratumoral temperature and higher tissue ablation volume in a shorter ablation cycle than RFA [5, 20–22].

2.5.5 Limitations/complications

It carries the risk of affecting the diagnostic accuracy of the cut edge [5].

2.6 Hydro-jet-assisted technique

2.6.1 Methods

Hydro-jet-assisted minimally invasive partial nephrectomy (MIPN) is performed by blunt dissection and dissection of the renal parenchyma using extremely thin, high-pressure water flow. The spread of tumor cells may be caused when hydro-jet dissection is performed for malignant diseases.

2.6.2 Results

Gao and colleagues performed hydro-jet-assisted minimally invasive partial nephrectomy.The average operation time was (103.2 ± 24.5)min, the average intraoperative blood loss was (250.3 ± 80.6) ml, the average perirenal drainage tube induration was (6.3 ± 2.6) days, and the average postoperative hospital stay was (8.3 ± 1.6) days [23].

2.6.3 Complications

The spread of tumor cells may be caused when hydro-jet dissection is performed for malignant diseases [24].

2.6.4 Advantages and limitations

Water jet uses the kinetic energy of water to separate the human tissue, without any thermal damage, and will not cause damage to the important organs and surrounding tissues [25]. Water jet, with high tissue selectivity and protection, can achieve the purpose of accurate protection of blood vessels, nerves, and canals and reduce the possibility of accidental injury [23].

However, compared with other methods, the cutting speed of water jet is relatively low. Meanwhile, in the process of cutting with water knife, a large amount of water waste liquid will be produced, which may affect the observation of surgical field and the judgment of cutting surface [11].

3. Introduction of unassisted zero-ischemia surgery

3.1 Unassisted zero-ischemia partial nephrectomy

3.1.1 Methods

To obtain a bloodless field and, consequently, to perform precise tumor excision and renal reconstruction, contemporary partial nephrectomy (PN) techniques typically need hilar clamping, which necessarily imposes ischemic and reperfusion injuries upon the kidney [26]. The unassisted zero-ischemia PN technique aims to reduce or even eliminate these injuries and preserves renal function [27].

In 2011, Gill et al. introduced "Zero-Ischemia" partial nephrectomy as a new technique to perform minimally invasive partial nephrectomy (MIPN) with selective renal artery clamping. Firstly, to precisely guide the clamping of tumor-supplying branches, the feeding branch for the tumor is identified by angiographic evaluation or computed tomography angiography (CTA). Then followed is the microdissection of renal arterial branches. The hilar vessels should be preemptively prepared before the meticulous microdissection and clip ligation of the tertiary or quaternary renal arterial branch which dedicatedly supplies the tumor or the tumor-bearing segment of the kidney [26]. Related clinical studies have been carried out and suggested that selective renal artery clamping can achieve no inferior or even better effect than hilar clamping [28, 29].

Though the selective clamping technique reduces the ischemic renal injury, the ischemic area of selective renal artery clamping is still larger than the tumor area. In addition, it is necessary to dissect tertiary or quaternary renal arteries, prolong the operation time, and increase the stimulation of renal arteries. PN without clamping any artery called off-clamping technique aims to optimize this short-coming. The operation is similar to on-clamping PN. The renal artery needs to be dissected and marked, but will not be clamped. Renal tumor and part of the kidney are dissected. Then the tumor is resected 0.5-1 cm away from the tumor edge without blocking the renal artery. The renal parenchyma is sutured continuously with inverted thorn thread, or bipolar electrocoagulation is given to stop bleeding and cover the hemostatic material. Drainage tube is indwelled after examination of no active bleeding [30].

3.1.2 Indications and contraindications

The indication for the application of zero-ischemia PN is not clear. Based on the indications and contraindications of on-clamping PN, the location, number, growth pattern (endogenous/exogenous), and intrarenal size of the tumor are the main factors to consider in operating this technique.

Zero-ischemia PN appears suited for medially located, whether in hilar, central, or polar sites. The medially located tumor or its bearing segment of the kidney is typically supplied by a dedicated secondary, tertiary, or quaternary branch [26]. However, tumors with dense or adherent perirenal fat or short segmental arteries may not be suggested to perform selective arterial clamping [31].

The application of off-clamping remains controversial. Whether under laparoscopic or robotic assist, unacceptable bleeding caused by off-clamping will lead to unclear visual field and difficult to complete high-precision surgery. Thus, off-clamping is limited to the tumors with favorably anatomical features (i.e. small, superficial, exophytic) and technically relatively easy [26].

3.1.3 Results and complications

The ideal goal of PN is to achieve Trifecta, that is, complete resection of the tumor ensures negative surgical margin, maximum preservation of normal nephron function, and avoidance of short-term and long-term complications. The negative surgical margin is the most important one [32].

In the study reported by GILL, SHAO, and NG, all patients who performed zero-ischemia PN achieve negative surgical margins [26, 28, 33]. In the study reported by SMITH and THOMPSON, the positive rate of tumor surgical margin is not significantly different between zero-ischemia PN and on-clamping PN [34, 35]. The study from WSZOLEK et al. tends to highly selective renal artery clamping can reduce the positive rate of the surgical margin, but the local recurrence rate and the 5-year survival rate in postoperative follow-up are similar [36].

Complications of zero-ischemia PN are similar to those of on-clamping PN due to the similar operation method. The study from WSZOLEK and THOMPSON revealed that on-clamping PN has a higher urine leakage rate and hemorrhage rate than zero-ischemia PN, but the results have no significant statistical significance [35, 36].

3.1.4 Advantages and limitations

That zero-ischemia PN is suited for anatomically favorable tumors results in on-clamping PN having a wider scope of application than zero-ischemia PN. During zero-ischemia PN, the increase in blood loss leads to unclear visual field and more difficult operation. The dissection of the tertiary or quaternary renal arterial branch prolongs the operation time.

But the ischemia time and area are reduced. It helps preserve more renal parenchyma and protects renal function. What's more, for patients with cardiovascular complications, potential renal dysfunction, or old age, ischemia may lead to greater injury, so zero-ischemia technology has a comparative advantage [26].

3.2 Unassisted zero-ischemia tumor enucleation

3.2.1 Methods

For zero-ischemia tumor enucleation (TE), retroperitoneal fashion is typically accepted. The location of the tumor is determined according to the preoperative imaging data. The main renal artery needs to be isolated routinely. The resection initiated approximately 2 mm away from the tumor margin. After identifying the pseudocapsule, the surgeon took the pseudocapsule as an anatomic marker to enucleate the tumor from the surface to the bottom using blunt together with sharp dissection [37].

3.2.2 Indications and contraindications

Similar to PN, TE is mainly suitable for patients with lateral exophytic tumors with early stage, especially T1 renal cell carcinoma, and requires that the tumor has a pseudocapsule that has not been breached. Thus, for the endogenous tumor, the large intrarenal tumor, and the tumor have breached the pseudocapsule, zero-ischemia tumor enucleation is not a suitable operation. In addition, the zero-ischemia technique should not be applied to patients with severe bleeding tendency or severe anemia. For T2 renal cell carcinoma, whether using this technique should base on the anatomical features and techniques of surgeons.

3.2.3 Results and complications

The curative effect of simple enucleation (SE) of renal tumors provides a reference for zero-ischemia tumor enucleation. For localized renal cell carcinoma, there is no significant difference in the positive rate of surgical margin, local recurrence rate, and survival rate between SE and PN [2]. Minervini reported a case of 127 patients who performed robot-assisted SE with a median follow-up of 61 months. There was no recurrence in situ [38]. The 10-year tumor-specific survival rate of SE was 97% [39].

Complications of zero-ischemia enucleation include postoperative bleeding, urinary fistula, short-term and long-term decline of renal function caused by reduced renal parenchyma, and postoperative infection.

3.2.4 Advantages and limitations

Compared with PN, TE preserves more renal parenchyma to ensure better renal function but has a smaller scope of application due to the oncological and anatomical requirements [37].

Compared with off-clamping TE, the incidence of CKD of zero-ischemia TE is lower [40], and the reduction rate of postoperative GFR is lower [28]. The indexes such as creatinine in the zero-ischemia TE are also better than those in off-clamping TE [18]. But the intraoperative blood loss was higher.

3.3 Sequential preplaced suture Renorrhaphy technique

3.3.1 Methods

The method of this surgery was firstly described in 2013 by Emad et al. [41]. It is roughly the same as minimally partial nephrectomy in the process before tumor resection. Notably, sequential preplaced suture renorrhaphy technique is to excise the renal tumor between the tumor edge and the suture replaced through the tissue adjacent to the tumor and modifying placement of the suture real time until the mass is completely excised.

3.3.2 Indications and contraindications

Similar to other zero-ischemia minimally invasive partial nephrectomy surgeries, sequential preplaced suture renorrhaphy technique is mostly applicable to patients who require eliminating warm ischemia urgently, such as those with solitary kidneys or multiple tumors. As for the size and location of the tumor, it is practical for treating RCCs with small tumor sizes, especially whose diameter is smaller than 3 cm and which are exophytic and peripheral renal tumors. In other words, this technique is limited for treating hilar located tumors.

3.3.3 Results and complications

The results of this surgery were not worse than other MIPNs. There did not exsit a statistically significant difference between preoperative and 12-month postoperative creatinine and eGFR values [42]. As shown in a previous study [41], median estimated blood loss (EBL) was 192.5 mL while median operative time was 160 minutes, which were similar to other zero-ischemia surgeries. What is more, according to the postoperative pathology findings in multiple investigations, almost all of the tumors treated with it had negative surgical margins and were completely eliminated. After the surgery, postoperative ileus, blood transfusion, and deep vein thrombosis were the main postoperative problems. Another study found the average operating duration was 75 minutes and a 60-ml average blood loss [43]. All 14 cases had negative surgical margins, and there was no postoperative bleeding or urine leakage after surgery. There were no signs of recurrence on a follow-up CT conducted 1–6 months after surgery. However, results of this surgery still need long-term follow-up.

DOI: http://dx.doi.org/10.5772/intechopen.109444

3.3.4 Advantages and limitations

Compared with other surgeries which need warm ischemia, it avoids renal ischemia reperfusion injury and preserves more renal function. Compared to other straightforward excision without hilar clamping, it improves visibility as a result of less bleeding and helps to excise less normal parenchyma and thereby minimize nephron loss. Moreover, suture placement can be more precisely adjusted in real time, which increases resection precision and lessens the likelihood of a positive margin.

The limited application of this method is to treat tumors with hilar locations. Besides, prepositioning the suture will compress and deform the tumor bed, making tumor removal challenging or erroneous. We still need more sample sizes and longer time to follow-up to verify its effectiveness and oncologic safety during the process of implementation [11].

4. Application of the three-dimensional visualization technology of renal vasculature

The arterial blood supply of renal cell carcinoma is diversified. Generally speaking, the main renal artery is the main blood supply artery for renal tumors. However, extrarenal blood supply arteries often participate in tumor angiogenesis, playing a very important role in tumor blood supply [44, 45]. Borojeni found that about 26 patients had multiple renal segmental arterial blood supply through renal arteriography of 60 patients with stage T1 renal carcinoma [46].

In recent years, with the development of minimally invasive technology and the implementation of the concept of "zero ischemia," laparoscopic partial nephrectomy more often uses selective renal artery clamping. High-selective clamping of the segmental artery which irrigated the tumor can not only obtain good effect of blocking tumor blood supply but also effectively reduce the renal warm ischemia time of patients and reduce the risk of surgery. Francesco Porpigilia et al. studied 52 cases of robot-assisted partial nephrectomy and showed that compared with the control group, the preoperative hyperaccuracy three-dimensional (HA3D) reconstruction technology can accurately display the course and surrounding structures of renal tumor-related renal segment branches, thus improving the success rate of clamping renal tumor-related renal artery branches during operation [6].

As an imaging tool of digital medical technology, three-dimensional visualization uses computer image processing technology to process CT or MRI image data through the workstation, import the data into the three-dimensional visualization imaging software system for segmentation, fusion, calculation, rendering and other operations, and build a three-dimensional model. The model can describe and explain the precise location, spatial anatomy, shape and volume of target lesions, related organs and vascular systems from multiple angles and in an all-round way and can provide clinicians with intuitive visual experience and full quantitative information. It is of high value for accurate preoperative diagnosis, planning of individualized surgical programs, and prediction of surgical risks. Further studies have shown that three-dimensional visualization can clearly display the number, size, branching pattern, shape, and positional relationship with renal tumors of the aberrant renal arteries, thereby helping the surgeon to determine the anatomical shape of renal blood vessels and the location of ectopic blood vessels before surgery and provide accurate guidance intraoperative operation [47].

5. Advances in renal carcinoma complexity scoring systems

Currently available nephrometry scores can arbitrarily be grouped into those based on a visual anatomical assessment of a renal mass and those based on a mathematical assessment.

Most of the scores are included in this group because they are based on an immediate visual evaluation. The RENAL and PADUA scores assess the location of the tumor, its percentage of penetration into the kidney, and its relationship with the renal sinus or urinary collecting system [48]. The Diameter-Axial-Polar (DAP) score determines the size of kidney mass and distance from two reference lines: axial and polar lines [49]. The Zonal Nearness-Physical-Radius Organization (NePhRO) score provides five parameters that mirror RENAL and PADUA scores. The difference is that it divides the kidney into three zones (zone 1: kidney parenchyma; zone 2: medullary and sinus; and zone 3: collecting system and hilum) and employs another dimensional scale to determine renal mass dimension [50]. Otherwise, the Renal Pelvic Score (RPS) deviates from the previously mentioned scores. Indeed, it evaluates the presence of an intrarenal or extrarenal pelvis referring to a sagittal line which passes through the kidney hilum [51]. The Surgical Approach Renal Ranking (SARR), a different score, has the same characteristics as the RENAL, PADUA, and Zonal NePhRO scores but offers a scoring system range from 0 to 4, rendering it possible to achieve a more precise stratification of renal masses [52]. The majority of scores take the tumor's longitudinal position into account; however, the Zhongshan score also takes into account the transversal tumor, which includes its lateral, central, and medial locations [53]. Recently, developments in the Simplified PAdua REnal (SPARE) nephrometry system has combined the key elements of both the nephrometry scores to create a maximum tumor size, exophytic rate, renal sinus involvement, and tumor rim location-based score [54]. The Arterial-Based Complexity (ABC) scoring system takes the order of vessels needed to be transected/dissected into account. The four scores (1, 2, 3S, and 3 H) evaluated are related to the neoplasm interaction with interlobular and arcuate arteries, interlobar arteries, segmental arteries, or in close proximity of the renal hilum, respectively [55]. The Peritumoral Artery Scoring System (PASS) is another score based on the vasculature [56]. Based on the number and diameter of the peritumoral arteries, this three-dimensional score assigns a complexity level to tumor dissection. The Mayo Adhesive Probability (MAP) score, in contrast to the scores stated above, assesses the perinephric fat thickness as a means to anticipate its adhesion to the kidney, which could result in a more complicated resection [57].

This category necessitates a thorough imaging examination and is based either on a mathematical or visual evaluation of the tumor. The first one, the Centrality Index (C-index), categorizes the complexity of the tumor according to the mathematical distance between the tumor and kidney center [58]. The Renal Tumor Invasion Index (RTII), which is the ratio of tumor invasion depth, is defined as the maximal distance that tumor invades into parenchyma and the parenchymal thickness of the kidney immediately adjacent to the tumor [59]. Both the tumor Contact Surface Area (CSA) and the Renal And Ischemia Volume (RAIV) use measurements of the mass radius and diameter. Additionally, the RAIV demands that the cross section of the resected and ischemized renal parenchyma be measured. [60, 61]. In a similar manner, the Zero Ischemia Index (ZII) shows the outcome of multiplying the tumor's depth in the kidney parenchyma by its diameter. [62]. The Coefficient,

Location, Anterior boundary, Multi-boundary, and Posterior boundary (CLAMP) score is the only used to determine the complexity of vascular. This three-dimensional (3D) imaging-based score assesses the anatomy of the arteries that supply the renal tumor. This instrument could estimate the effectiveness of segmental artery clamping [62].

The Mayo Clinic thrombus classification is widely used to describe levels of inferior vena cava tumor thrombus and is significant to guide the operation for renal cell carcinoma with venous thrombus in the open era [7]. But in the minimally invasive surgery era, Prof. Zhang et al. summarized a large number of surgical experiences of renal cell carcinoma with venous thrombus and put forward the "301 classification" system. The system based on anatomical landmarks in which one grade corresponds to one surgical strategy improves surgical choice in the treatment of renal cell carcinoma with venous thrombus. The right renal vein tumor thrombus was Level 0, and the surgical strategy was radical resection of the right kidney; left renal vein tumor thrombus can be divided into Level 0a and 0b according to whether it exceeds the superior mesenteric artery [8]. In 0a, radical resection of the left kidney is performed. In 0b, left renal artery embolism is performed before operation. First, the left renal vein and inferior vena cava are disconnected in the left lateral position, and then radical resection of the left kidney is performed in a different position. The inferior vena cava tumor thrombus below the first porta hepatis was level I, which did not need to turn over the liver, only needed to lift the liver and cut off 1–3 short hepatic veins. The level from the first porta hepatis to the second porta hepatis is level II, and it is necessary to turn the right hepatic lobe, without blocking the hepatic blood flow, and disconnect 2 to 5 short hepatic veins. The level from the second hepatic portal to the diaphragm is Level III, which requires turning the left and right hepatic lobes, and blocking the portal blood flow. During the operation, venous-venous bypass is performed according to the situation, and more short hepatic veins are cut off; Level IV is above the diaphragm [63]. Cardiopulmonary extracorporeal circulation should be established to block the superior vena cava and the inferior vena cava above the diaphragm. Thoracoscopic surgery should be performed to remove the atrial tumor thrombus and then block the hepatic portal vessels, and the distal inferior vena cava and its branches. For level 0 or 0a tumor thrombus, laparoscopic surgery is the first choice. For 0b or inferior vena cava tumor thrombus, robotic surgery is the first choice. If the tumor is large, has a complex surgical history, and the function of organs such as the heart is not complete, and it is necessary to shorten the operation time or establish venous bypass, open surgery is the first choice.

6. Conclusion

Most cases of RCC have no clinical symptoms but are diagnosed accidentally. With the development of diagnostic technology, the incidence of patients diagnosed with RCC has increased rapidly over the past decades. For the majority of patients diagnosed with RCC, choosing the appropriate treatment is the primary means to improve their prognosis. Therefore, knowing the latest surgical progress and being familiar with the renal carcinoma complexity scoring system could help doctors design more individualized and appropriate surgical procedures for patients, allowing surgeons to preserve more renal parenchyma while fully removing the tumor.

Author details

Congcong Xu[1], Dekai Liu[2], Chengcheng Xing[2], Jiaqi Du[2], Gangfu Zheng[2], Nengfeng Yu[2], Dingya Zhou[2], Honghui Cheng[2], Kefan Yang[2], Qifeng Zhong[2] and Yichun Zheng[1,2*]

1 The Second Affiliated Hospital, Zhejiang University School of Medicine, Hangzhou, China

2 The Fourth Affiliated Hospital, Zhejiang University School of Medicine, Yiwu, China

*Address all correspondence to: 2101090@zju.edu.cn

References

[1] Escudier B, Porta C, Schmidinger M, et al. Renal cell carcinoma: ESMO clinical practice guidelines for diagnosis, treatment and follow-up†. Annals of Oncology. 2019;**30**(5):706-720. Epub 2019/02/23. DOI: 10.1093/annonc/mdz056

[2] Xu C, Lin C, Xu Z, Feng S, Zheng Y. Tumor enucleation vs. partial nephrectomy for T1 renal cell carcinoma: A systematic review and meta-analysis. Frontiers in Oncology. 2019;**9**:473. Epub 2019/06/20. DOI: 10.3389/fonc.2019.00473

[3] Ljungberg B, Albiges L, Abu-Ghanem Y, et al. European Association of Urology guidelines on renal cell carcinoma: The 2022 update. European Urology. 2022;**82**(4):399-410. Epub 2022/03/30. DOI: 10.1016/j.eururo.2022.03.006

[4] Campbell S, Uzzo RG, Allaf ME, et al. Renal mass and localized renal cancer: AUA guideline. The Journal of Urology. 2017;**198**(3):520-529. Epub 2017/05/10. DOI: 10.1016/j.juro.2017.04.100

[5] Zhou J, Wu X, Zhang J, Huang J, Chen Y. Mid-to-long term oncologic and functional outcomes of zero ischemia laparoscopic microwave ablation-assisted tumor enucleation for renal cell carcinoma: A single-center experience. Translational Cancer Research. 2021;**10**(5):2328-2336. Epub 2022/02/05. DOI: 10.21037/tcr-20-2846

[6] Porpiglia F, Fiori C, Checcucci E, Amparore D, Bertolo R. Hyperaccuracy three-dimensional reconstruction is able to maximize the efficacy of selective clamping during robot-assisted partial nephrectomy for complex renal masses. European Urology. 2018;**74**(5):651-660. Epub 2018/01/11. DOI: 10.1016/j.eururo.2017.12.027

[7] Blute ML, Leibovich BC, Lohse CM, Cheville JC, Zincke H. The Mayo Clinic experience with surgical management, complications and outcome for patients with renal cell carcinoma and venous tumour thrombus. BJU International. 2004;**94**(1):33-41. Epub 2004/06/26. DOI: 10.1111/j.1464-410X.2004.04897.x

[8] Wang B, Li H, Ma X, et al. Robot-assisted laparoscopic inferior vena cava Thrombectomy: Different sides require different techniques. European Urology. 2016;**69**(6):1112-1119. Epub 2015/12/27. DOI: 10.1016/j.eururo.2015.12.001

[9] Simone G, Papalia R, Guaglianone S, Forestiere E, Gallucci M. Preoperative superselective transarterial embolization in laparoscopic partial nephrectomy: Technique, oncologic, and functional outcomes. Journal of Endourology. 2009;**23**(9):1473-1478. Epub 2009/08/22. DOI: 10.1089/end.2009.0334

[10] D'Urso L, Simone G, Rosso R, et al. Benefits and shortcomings of superselective transarterial embolization of renal tumors before zero ischemia laparoscopic partial nephrectomy. European Journal of Surgical Oncology. 2014;**40**(12):1731-1737. Epub 2014/10/08. DOI: 10.1016/j.ejso.2014.08.484

[11] Hou W, Ji Z. Achieving zero ischemia in minimally invasive partial nephrectomy surgery. International Journal of Surgery. 2015;**18**:48-54. Epub 2015/04/22. DOI: 10.1016/j.ijsu.2015.04.046

[12] Nohara T, Fujita H, Yamamoto K, Kitagawa Y, Gabata T, Namiki M. Modified anatrophic partial nephrectomy

with selective renal segmental artery clamping to preserve renal function: A preliminary report. International Journal of Urology. 2008;**15**(11):961-966. Epub 2008/09/24. DOI: 10.1111/j.1442-2042.2008.02141.x

[13] Wang CH, Li CS, Jiang Y, Zhang H, Mu HD, Bao GC. The efficacy evaluation of partial nephrectomy with selective renal artery branch occlusion by laparoscopy. Medicine (Baltimore). 2021;**100**(26):e26581. Epub 2021/07/01. DOI: 10.1097/md.0000000000026581

[14] Thomas AZ, Smyth L, Hennessey D, O'Kelly F, Moran D, Lynch TH. Zero ischemia laparoscopic partial thulium laser nephrectomy. Journal of Endourology. 2013;**27**(11):1366-1370. Epub 2013/01/11. DOI: 10.1089/end.2012.0527

[15] Wang Y, Shao J, Lü Y, Li X. Thulium laser-assisted versus conventional laparoscopic partial nephrectomy for the small renal mass. Lasers in Surgery and Medicine. 2020;**52**(5):402-407. Epub 2019/09/05. DOI: 10.1002/lsm.23153

[16] Kyriazis I, Ozsoy M, Kallidonis P, Panagopoulos V, Vasilas M, Liatsikos E. Current evidence on lasers in laparoscopy: Partial nephrectomy. World Journal of Urology. 2015;**33**(4):589-594. Epub 2014/07/06. DOI: 10.1007/s00345-014-1343-0

[17] Zhao X, Zhang S, Liu G, et al. Zero ischemia laparoscopic radio frequency ablation assisted enucleation of renal cell carcinoma: Experience with 42 patients. The Journal of Urology. 2012;**188**(4):1095-1101. Epub 2012/08/21. DOI: 10.1016/j.juro.2012.06.035

[18] Zhang C, Zhao X, Guo S, Ji C, Wang W, Guo H. Perioperative outcomes of zero ischemia radiofrequency ablation-assisted tumor enucleation for renal cell carcinoma: Results of 182 patients. BMC Urology. 2018;**18**(1):41. Epub 2018/05/17. DOI: 10.1186/s12894-018-0356-1

[19] Huang J, Zhang J, Wang Y, et al. Comparing zero ischemia laparoscopic radio frequency ablation assisted tumor enucleation and laparoscopic partial nephrectomy for clinical T1a renal tumor: A randomized clinical trial. The Journal of Urology. 2016;**195**(6):1677-1683. Epub 2016/02/26. DOI: 10.1016/j.juro.2015.12.115

[20] Wilcox Vanden Berg RN, Calderon LP. LaRussa S, et al. microwave ablation of cT1a renal cell carcinoma: Oncologic and functional outcomes at a single center. Clinical Imaging. 2021;**76**:199-204. Epub 2021/05/09. DOI: 10.1016/j.clinimag.2021.04.016

[21] Moinzadeh A, Gill IS, Finelli A, Kaouk J, Desai M. Laparoscopic partial nephrectomy: 3-year followup. The Journal of Urology. 2006;**175**(2):459-462. Epub 2006/01/13. DOI: 10.1016/s0022-5347(05)00147-3

[22] McCarthy CJ, Gervais DA. Decision making: Thermal ablation options for small renal masses. Seminars in Interventional Radiology. 2017;**34**(2):167-175. Epub 2017/06/06. DOI: 10.1055/s-0037-1602708

[23] Shekarriz B. Hydro-jet technology in urologic surgery. Expert Review of Medical Devices. 2005;**2**(3):287-291. Epub 2005/11/18. DOI: 10.1586/17434440.2.3.287

[24] Gao Y, Chen L, Ning Y, et al. Hydro-jet-assisted laparoscopic partial nephrectomy with no renal arterial clamping: A preliminary study in a single center. International Urology and Nephrology. 2014;**46**(7):1289-1293. Epub 2014/03/19. DOI: 10.1007/s11255-014-0670-9

[25] Osman Y, Harraz AM. A review comparing experience and results with bipolar versus monopolar resection for treatment of bladder tumors. Current Urology Reports. 2016;**17**(3):21. Epub 2016/02/16. DOI: 10.1007/s11934-016-0579-1

[26] Gill IS, Eisenberg MS, Aron M, et al. "zero ischemia" partial nephrectomy: Novel laparoscopic and robotic technique. European Urology. 2011;**59**(1):128-134. Epub 2010/10/26. DOI: 10.1016/j.eururo.2010.10.002

[27] Wszolek MF, Kenney PA, Libertino JA. Nonclamping partial nephrectomy: Towards improved nephron sparing. Nature Reviews. Urology. 2011;**8**(9):523-527. Epub 2011/08/04. DOI: 10.1038/nrurol.2011.103

[28] Shao P, Qin C, Yin C, et al. Laparoscopic partial nephrectomy with segmental renal artery clamping: Technique and clinical outcomes. European Urology. 2011;**59**(5):849-855. Epub 2010/12/15. DOI: 10.1016/j.eururo.2010.11.037

[29] Desai MM, de Castro Abreu AL, Leslie S, et al. Robotic partial nephrectomy with superselective versus main artery clamping: A retrospective comparison. European Urology. 2014;**66**(4):713-719. Epub 2014/02/04. DOI: 10.1016/j.eururo.2014.01.017

[30] Wu SD, Viprakasit DP, Cashy J, Smith ND, Perry KT, Nadler RB. Radiofrequency ablation-assisted robotic laparoscopic partial nephrectomy without renal hilar vessel clamping versus laparoscopic partial nephrectomy: A comparison of perioperative outcomes. Journal of Endourology. 2010;**24**(3):385-391. Epub 2010/03/26. DOI: 10.1089/end.2009.0199

[31] Klatte T, Ficarra V, Gratzke C, et al. A literature review of renal surgical anatomy and surgical strategies for partial nephrectomy. European Urology. 2015;**68**(6):980-992. Epub 2015/04/26. DOI: 10.1016/j.eururo.2015.04.010

[32] Shah PH, Moreira DM, Okhunov Z, et al. Positive surgical margins increase risk of recurrence after partial nephrectomy for high risk renal tumors. The Journal of Urology. 2016;**196**(2):327-334. Epub 2016/02/26. DOI: 10.1016/j.juro.2016.02.075

[33] Ng CK, Gill IS, Patil MB, et al. Anatomic renal artery branch microdissection to facilitate zero-ischemia partial nephrectomy. European Urology. 2012;**61**(1):67-74. Epub 2011/09/13. DOI: 10.1016/j.eururo.2011.08.040

[34] Smith GL, Kenney PA, Lee Y, Libertino JA. Non-clamped partial nephrectomy: Techniques and surgical outcomes. BJU International. 2011;**107**(7):1054-1058. Epub 2010/11/03. DOI: 10.1111/j.1464-410X.2010.09798.x

[35] Thompson RH, Lane BR, Lohse CM, et al. Every minute counts when the renal hilum is clamped during partial nephrectomy. European Urology. 2010;**58**(3):340-345. Epub 2010/09/10. DOI: 10.1016/j.eururo.2010.05.047

[36] Wszolek MF, Kenney PA, Lee Y, Libertino JA. Comparison of hilar clamping and non-hilar clamping partial nephrectomy for tumours involving a solitary kidney. BJU International. 2011;**107**(12):1886-1892. Epub 2010/11/13. DOI: 10.1111/j.1464-410X.2010.09713.x

[37] Dell'Atti L, Scarcella S, Manno S, Polito M, Galosi AB. Approach for renal tumors with low Nephrometry score through unclamped Sutureless

laparoscopic enucleation technique: Functional and oncologic outcomes. Clinical Genitourinary Cancer. 2018;**16**(6):e1251-e12e6. Epub 2018/08/21. DOI: 10.1016/j.clgc.2018.07.020

[38] Minervini A, Campi R, Di Maida F, et al. Tumor-parenchyma interface and long-term oncologic outcomes after robotic tumor enucleation for sporadic renal cell carcinoma. Urologic Oncology. 2018;**36**(12):527.e1-527e11. Epub 2018/10/01. DOI: 10.1016/j.urolonc.2018.08.014

[39] Singer EA, Vourganti S, Lin KY, et al. Outcomes of patients with surgically treated bilateral renal masses and a minimum of 10 years of followup. The Journal of Urology. 2012;**188**(6):2084-2088. Epub 2012/10/23. DOI: 10.1016/j.juro.2012.08.038

[40] Kopp RP, Mehrazin R, Palazzi K, Bazzi WM, Patterson AL, Derweesh IH. Factors affecting renal function after open partial nephrectomy-a comparison of clampless and clamped warm ischemic technique. Urology. 2012;**80**(4):865-870. Epub 2012/09/07. DOI: 10.1016/j.urology.2012.04.079

[41] Rizkala ER, Khalifeh A, Autorino R, Samarasekera D, Laydner H, Kaouk JH. Zero ischemia robotic partial nephrectomy: Sequential preplaced suture renorrhaphy technique. Urology. 2013;**82**(1):100-104. Epub 2013/06/29. DOI: 10.1016/j.urology.2013.03.042

[42] Sönmez MG, Kara C. The effect of zero-ischaemia laparoscopic minimally invasive partial nephrectomy using the modified sequential preplaced suture renorrhaphy technique on long-term renal functions. Wideochir Inne Tech Maloinwazyjne. 2017;**12**(3):257-263. Epub 2017/10/25. DOI: 10.5114/wiitm.2017.67136

[43] Lu J, Zu Q, Du Q, Xu Y, Zhang X, Dong J. Zero ischaemia laparoscopic nephron-sparing surgery by re-suturing. Contemporay Oncology (Pozn). 2014;**18**(5):355-358. Epub 2014/12/06. DOI: 10.5114/wo.2014.41385

[44] Brindle MJ. Alternative vascular channels in renal cell carcinoma. Clinical Radiology. 1972;**23**(3):321-330. Epub 1972/07/01. DOI: 10.1016/s0009-9260(72)80058-8

[45] Sprayregen S. Parasitic blood supply of neoplasms. Mechanisms and significance. Radiology. 1973;**106**(3):529-535. Epub 1973/03/01. DOI: 10.1148/106.3.529

[46] Borojeni S, Borojeni A, Panayotopoulos P, et al. Study of renal and kidney tumor vascularization using data from preoperative three-dimensional arteriography prior to partial nephrectomy. European Urology Focus. 2020;**6**(1):112-121. Epub 2018/08/07. DOI: 10.1016/j.euf.2018.07.028

[47] Porpiglia F, Checcucci E, Amparore D, et al. Three-dimensional augmented reality robot-assisted partial nephrectomy in case of complex Tumours (PADUA ≥10): A new intraoperative tool overcoming the ultrasound guidance. European Urology. 2020;**78**(2):229-238. Epub 2020/01/04. DOI: 10.1016/j.eururo.2019.11.024

[48] Kutikov A, Uzzo RG. The R.E.N.a.L. nephrometry score: A comprehensive standardized system for quantitating renal tumor size, location and depth. The Journal of Urology. 2009;**182**(3):844-853. Epub 2009/07/21. DOI: 10.1016/j.juro.2009.05.035

[49] Simmons MN, Hillyer SP, Lee BH, Fergany AF, Kaouk J, Campbell SC. Diameter-axial-polar nephrometry:

Integration and optimization of R.E.N.a.L. and centrality index scoring systems. The Journal of Urology. 2012;**188**(2):384-390. Epub 2012/06/16. DOI: 10.1016/j.juro.2012.03.123

[50] Hakky TS, Baumgarten AS, Allen B, et al. Zonal NePhRO scoring system: A superior renal tumor complexity classification model. Clinical Genitourinary Cancer. 2014;**12**(1):e13-e18. Epub 2013/10/15. DOI: 10.1016/j.clgc.2013.07.009

[51] Tomaszewski JJ, Cung B, Smaldone MC, et al. Renal pelvic anatomy is associated with incidence, grade, and need for intervention for urine leak following partial nephrectomy. European Urology. 2014;**66**(5):949-955. Epub 2013/11/05. DOI: 10.1016/j.eururo.2013.10.009

[52] Tannus M, Goldman SM, Andreoni C. Practical and intuitive surgical approach renal ranking to predict outcomes in the management of renal tumors: A novel score tool. Journal of Endourology. 2014;**28**(4):487-492. Epub 2014/01/21. DOI: 10.1089/end.2013.0148

[53] Zhou L, Guo J, Wang H, Wang G. The Zhongshan score: A novel and simple anatomic classification system to predict perioperative outcomes of nephron-sparing surgery. Medicine (Baltimore). 2015;**94**(5):e506. Epub 2015/02/06. DOI: 10.1097/md.0000000000000506

[54] Ficarra V, Porpiglia F, Crestani A, et al. The simplified PADUA REnal (SPARE) nephrometry system: A novel classification of parenchymal renal tumours suitable for partial nephrectomy. BJU International. 2019;**124**(4):621-628. DOI: 10.1111/bju.14772

[55] Spaliviero M, Poon BY, Karlo CA, et al. An arterial based complexity (ABC) scoring system to assess the morbidity profile of partial nephrectomy. European Urology. 2016;**69**(1):72-79. Epub 2015/08/25. DOI: 10.1016/j.eururo.2015.08.008

[56] Zhang R, Wu G, Huang J, et al. Peritumoral artery scoring system: A novel scoring system to predict renal function outcome after laparoscopic partial nephrectomy. Scientific Reports. 2017;**7**(1):2853. Epub 2017/06/08. DOI: 10.1038/s41598-017-03135-8

[57] Davidiuk AJ, Parker AS, Thomas CS, et al. Mayo adhesive probability score: An accurate image-based scoring system to predict adherent perinephric fat in partial nephrectomy. European Urology. 2014;**66**(6):1165-1171. Epub 2014/09/07. DOI: 10.1016/j.eururo.2014.08.054

[58] Simmons MN, Ching CB, Samplaski MK, Park CH, Gill IS. Kidney tumor location measurement using the C index method. The Journal of Urology. 2010;**183**(5):1708-1713. Epub 2010/03/20. DOI: 10.1016/j.juro.2010.01.005

[59] Nisen H, Ruutu M, Glücker E, Visapää H, Taari K. Renal tumour invasion index as a novel anatomical classification predicting urological complications after partial nephrectomy. Scandinavian Journal of Urology. 2014;**48**(1):41-51. Epub 2013/06/21. DOI: 10.3109/21681805.2013.797491

[60] Leslie S, Gill IS, de Castro Abreu AL, et al. Renal tumor contact surface area: A novel parameter for predicting complexity and outcomes of partial nephrectomy. European Urology. 2014;**66**(5):884-893. Epub 2014/04/01. DOI: 10.1016/j.eururo.2014.03.010

[61] Shin TY, Komninos C, Kim DW, et al. A novel mathematical model to predict the severity of postoperative functional reduction before partial nephrectomy:

The importance of calculating resected and ischemic volume. The Journal of Urology. 2015;**193**(2):423-429. Epub 2014/07/27. DOI: 10.1016/j.juro.2014.07.084

[62] Li Y, Zhou L, Bian T, et al. The zero ischemia index (ZII): A novel criterion for predicting complexity and outcomes of off-clamp partial nephrectomy. World Journal of Urology. 2017;**35**(7):1095-1102. Epub 2016/11/26. DOI: 10.1007/s00345-016-1975-3

[63] Wang B, Li H, Huang Q, et al. Robot-assisted Retrohepatic inferior vena cava Thrombectomy: First or second Porta Hepatis as an important boundary landmark. European Urology. 2018;**74**(4):512-520. Epub 2017/12/11. DOI: 10.1016/j.eururo.2017.11.017

Section 3

Imaging for Renal Cell Carcinoma

Chapter 6

Current Imaging Techniques in Renal Cell Carcinoma

Vaidehi Alpesh Patel

Abstract

Renal cancers are one of the 10 most commonly seen cancers in both sexes. The incidence of renal cancers is high in Western developed countries and lower in Eastern and developing countries. The overall incidence of malignancy has been increasing in recent times. Ultrasound (USG) is very commonly used imaging technique; however recent advances like contrast enhanced ultrasound helps to differentiate various cystic renal masses. Availability of newer imaging techniques such as Computed tomography scan (CT scan) and Magnetic resonance imaging (MRI) and their various applications may play a role in better and early diagnosis of such lesions. Due to its highly metastatic nature, accurate staging is more important to facilitate proper treatment. Fluoro-deoxyglucose positron emission tomography (FDG PET) is widely applied in detection, staging/restaging and surveillance of such lesions. In this chapter, we will try to cover the recent advances in various modalities for detection of renal cancers, particularly renal cell carcinoma (RCC).

Keywords: renal cancer, renal cell carcinoma, ultrasound, CT scan, MRI, PET scan, contrast enhanced ultrasound

1. Introduction

Renal cell carcinoma is the most common renal malignancy. The steady increase in incidental diagnosis of small renal cancers in last several decades can partly be dedicated to frequent abdominal imaging [1]. The risk benefit ratio has to be considered while resecting a renal mass for the presumption of cancer which can turn out to be of benign or indolent nature. Per cutaneous renal biopsy can be the gold standard for such pre surgical diagnosis; however it yields non diagnostic rate of 10–15% and the intra tumoral heterogeneity hampers its widespread use [1]. Hence, accurate pre surgical characterization of renal cancers is very needful to avoid over treatment and to facilitate the proper line of treatment to the surgeon.

Ultrasound is the most basic and commonly used imaging technique for diagnosis of renal cancers. It is non invasive, cost effective, readily available and widely used technique with advantages of real time imaging and without need of ionizing radiation. The basic disadvantage of USG is its operator dependency. Though USG is sufficient to differentiate simple or minimally complex cystic masses as benign lesions, it is not reliable to differentiate more complex cystic and solid lesions [1]. Newer advances in USG like contrast enhanced Ultrasound, ultrasound molecular imaging, elastography and micro doppler techniques are nowadays being investigated for better accuracy of ultrasound and to expand its role in tumor characterization.

Contrast enhanced CT scan (CECT) is considered the gold standard for the assessment of solid renal masses. CT scan offers the best imaging technique to properly diagnose and stage renal cell carcinoma along with post treatment surveillance. Post contrast mass enhancement and heterogeneous nature of renal masses also help to differentiate various subtypes of renal cell carcinoma but with less success. Apparent diffusion coefficient (ADC) distribution parameters for renal whole tumor are useful in discriminating oncocytoma from RCC [2]. Another pre processing method called Laplace of Gaussian (LoG) can be used to reduce the image noise while highlighting the degree of heterogeneity within the tumor and entropy can be used to quantify tumor heterogeneity. Both of these methods can be applied to conventional CT scan and can help substantially to predict the Fuhrman Grade of RCC [3].

Multi parametric MRI (mpMRI) is routinely used in clinical practice for renal mass evaluation nowadays. Common subtypes of RCC and other commonly seen benign epithelial renal masses can be non-invasively differentiated with the help of mpMRI. Recent advancement in algorithm for interpretation of mpMRI known as clear cell likelihood score (ccLS) can predict clear cell histology in cT1a mass. However it does not allow for prediction of high grade histology [4]. Another application is MR texture analysis (MRTA) which can generate several parameters showing excellent diagnostic value in differentiation of RCC from lipid poor angiomyolipoma (AML) and oncocytoma [5]. Contrast enhanced MRI (CEMRI) provides superior soft tissue resolution and delineates primary extent of tumor and venous tumor thrombus involvement. It is also useful for patients with iodine contrast allergies or in patients with impaired renal function. CEMRI can help in differentiation of tumor subtypes depending upon enhancement mode and apparent diffusion coefficient (ADC) values [6].

PET/CT scan simultaneously evaluates the lesion anatomy and provides metabolic information. It is widely used for pre operative staging and post operative restaging. Diagnostic results of primary RCC with FDG PET scan varies depending upon the tumor pathology and nuclear differentiation. FDG PET/CT detects venous tumor thrombus and can distinguish it from venous bland thrombus almost comparable to CEMRI. However PET/CT is more useful for distant organ metastasis [6]. Newer radio tracers like Prostate Specific Membrane Antigen (PSMA) also offer valid imaging option for RCC. Undefined renal mass evaluation and therapy response assessment can also be done with PSMA PET scan. PSMA based Radio ligand therapy is also a future development option. Recent advances like PET/MRI provide combined anatomic and metabolic information. It has very promising results in detection of RCC. However, detailed studies are in progress for its application.

2. Role of different imaging modalities in diagnosis of RCC

Role of Imaging in evaluation of RCC is for characterization of renal lesions. Various imaging modalities are being used for detailed evaluation of RCC in pre operative as well as post operative periods and also for guiding the proper treatment method along with for surveillance of RCC.

The first step in the process is to determine whether the lesion is cystic or solid. Cystic lesions are classified depending upon their imaging appearance using Bosniak classification system (**Table 1**). USG can easily describe these findings; however more complex and higher grade cysts need to be evaluated with further investigations. Solid

Category	Characteristics	Presentation
I	• Benign, simple cyst with well defined thin smooth wall (≤2 mm). • No evidence of septa, calcification or solid nodules. • Attenuation of contents equivalent to simple fluid (−9 to 20 HU) on unenhanced CT scan. • The wall may enhance on contrast studies.	
II	• Thin & smooth walls. • Few internal septa which can enhance. • May show wall calcification foci. • Homogeneous mass with −9 to 20 HU density on unenhanced CT scan. • Homogeneous hyper attenuating (≥70 HU) masses on unenhanced CT scan. • Homogeneous low attenuation masses that are too small to characterize.	
IIF	• Minimally thick (3 mm) smooth enhancing wall or septa or many (≥ 4 in number) thin (≤2 mm) enhancing septa. • Septal calcification focus	
III	• cystic masses with thick(≥4 mm width) irregular septa or smooth walls • septa with measurable enhancement	
IV	• clearly malignant cystic mass with criteria of category III • Also contains enhancing soft tissue components (≥4 mm) independent of wall or septa.	

Table 1.
Bosniak categorization criteria of renal masses with graphical presentation [7].

lesions can be accurately diagnosed as benign or malignant on the basis of CT or MRI findings. Once the lesion is diagnosed as solid or complex cystic lesion and the probability of RCC is made, further imaging plays an important role. In this section, we will cover the basic imaging features of RCC with various advances in each modality.

2.1 Ultrasound

Ultrasound (USG) is the basic investigation used to differentiate various renal cysts/masses. It is non invasive, readily available, cost effective imaging technique which offers real time imaging without risk of ionizing radiation. However major drawback of USG is its operator dependency. Conventional USG is capable to classify indeterminate renal masses with simple or minimally complex features as benign. However it is not reliable to classify more complex cystic or solid masses. The renal masses are characterized depending upon their walls and contents on USG and their various enhancement patterns on CT scan. Widely used classification method is Bosniak classification which includes various parameters like, cyst wall, internal septa (thickness and number) and their enhancement patterns, wall or septal calcifications, internal nodules and their enhancement (**Table 1**) [7]. Considerable proportion of renal masses may display equivocal features on Conventional CT scan and MRI which makes them difficult to be distinguished as benign or malignant [8]. Hence, various advancements are available or being studied for the non invasive use of USG in characterization of renal masses as follows.

2.1.1 Contrast enhanced ultrasound

Contrast enhanced ultrasound (CEUS) is newer technology addressing some of the drawbacks of non enhanced gray scale imaging and traditional color doppler ultrasound for evaluation of vascularization within the normal soft tissue or any focal lesion. Most commonly used contrast medium for CEUS is intravenously injectable micro bubbles. They are microspheres measuring about the size of red blood cells with biodegradable lipid or protein shell and a gas core. They are usually filled with per fluorocarbon like per flourobutane gas as it is heavier than air (for stability purpose). Other components like polyethylene glycol, proteins can also be added to the outer shell for improved stability.

Due to micron size of these bubbles (1–4 micrometer) they stay confined to the vessel and they can also pass through tiny capillaries. It enables high reflection and sound scatter in blood and they resonate non-linearly when insonnated by ultrasound waves. The unique signals gained from these micro bubbles are separated from the background which allows detection of blood flow within the tissue (**Figure 1**). The micro bubbles remain within the circulation for only few minutes and rapidly get cleared via reticulo-endothelial system and through lungs. Major advantage of ultrasound contrast agents over CT or MRI contrast agents is their use in renal insufficiency. First pass (bolus) dose of micro bubbles within the region of interest is done to assess levels of vascularity in real time with use of techniques like time intensity curve analysis, maximum intensity projection analysis or re-perfusion analysis. Contrast micro bubbles allow for better focal lesion detection and help to differentiate benign from malignant lesions. It also allows to measure tumor size accurately [8]. While lack of radiation, lower cost and high safety of contrast media are major advantages of CEUS, operator dependency and few other technical limitations are disadvantages of it which can limit its reproducibility.

Simple renal cyst shows no evidence of enhancement due to its clear contents and no vascularity within it. However, confusion due to equivocal findings for lower degree complex cysts can also be cleared with CEUS as many times a more complex cyst may not show enhancing contents on contrast scan and thus it can be stamped as

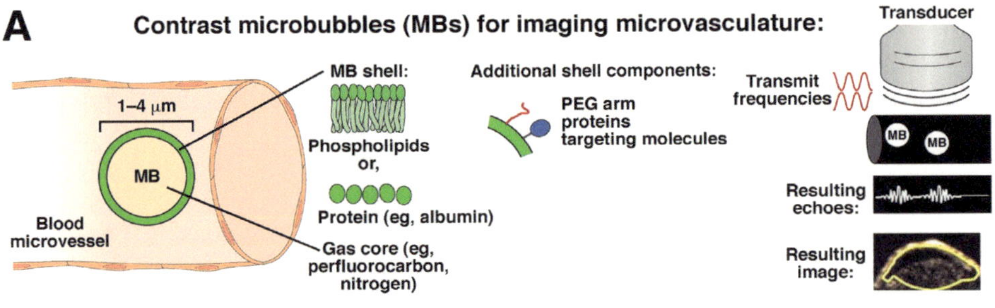

Figure 1.
Non targeted and molecularly targeted CEUS with micro bubbles. The gas core with shell of lipid or protein is basic formation of micro bubble (on left side). Pulse inversion technique is used for detection of micro bubbles. Two inverse phase (red colored) pulses are transmitted through the tissue and echoes are reflected back from micro bubbles or from tissue. The echo reflected from micro bubble represents white wave and from tissue represents flat line [8].

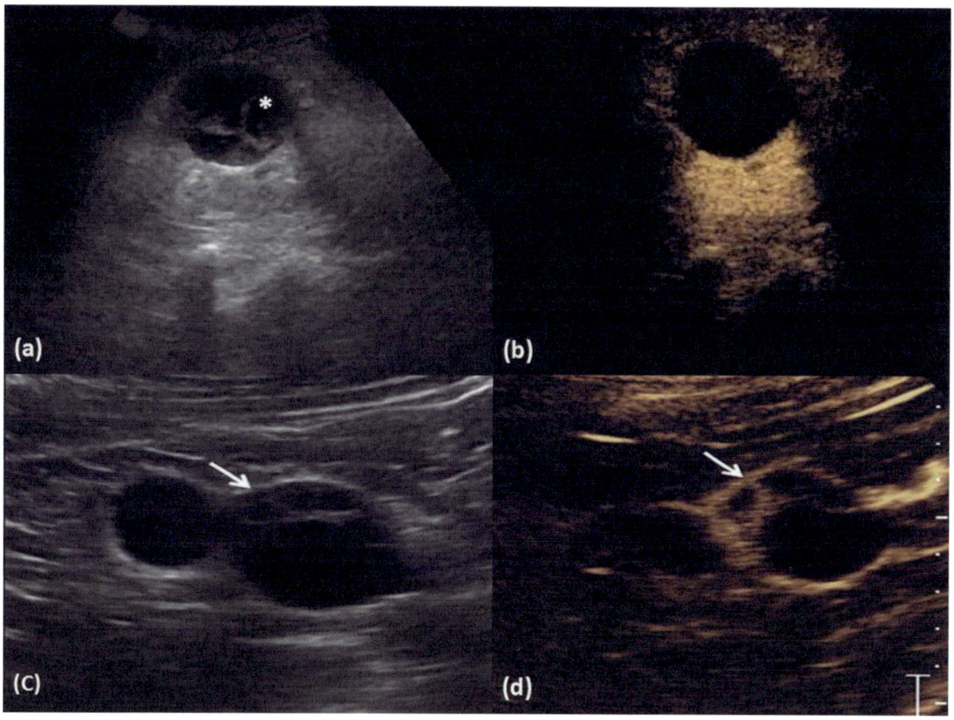

Figure 2.
(a) Gray scale imaging of renal cyst with internal thick septa (*). (b) on CEUS, the septa are not visible and the cyst remains clear. Final diagnosis is simple cyst. (c) Gray scale imaging of renal cyst with internal septa(white arrow) (d) on CEUS the internal septa enhance suggesting the cyst to be complex in nature [9].

benign lesion (**Figure 2**). Difference of perfusion within the lesion and surrounding renal cortex helps to characterize solid lesions also [1].

CEUS shows great value in evaluation of septations and mural nodules within the renal cysts due to their distinct enhancement. Equivocal results in Bosniak Category IIF and III cysts can be avoided with the use of CEUS. According to some studies CEUS has comparable results in classification of benign versus malignant renal masses as in CECT or CEMRI. According to Furrer et al., reported pooled sensitivity and specificity for CEUS, CECT and CEMRI in evaluation of renal masses to be 96%, 90% and 96% and 78%, 77% and 75% respectively [10]. Other researchers also compared CEUS with CECT and CEUS to CEMRI in solid renal lesions and reported almost similar results [11, 12]. However, lesions with fat within were excluded from these studies. Fat poor angiomyolipoma (AML) and oncocytoma have non differing imaging features on USG hence, they cannot be properly distinguished from RCC through CEUS. Quantitative features of CEUS i.e. analysis of time intensity curves help in distinction of various subtypes of RCC and from typical AML from RCC. However, there is considerable overlap in imaging features of these masses [1].

The enhancement of tumor less than that of surrounding renal parenchyma indicates it to be indolent or benign. However some benign lesions like oncocytoma also show hyper enhancement making it difficult to differentiate it from RCC on CEUS. However, RCC exhibits delayed contrast washout compared to adjacent renal parenchyma [13]. Marked enhancement and delayed washout of contrast medium are findings associated with clear cell RCC (ccRCC) (**Figure 3**). However these features

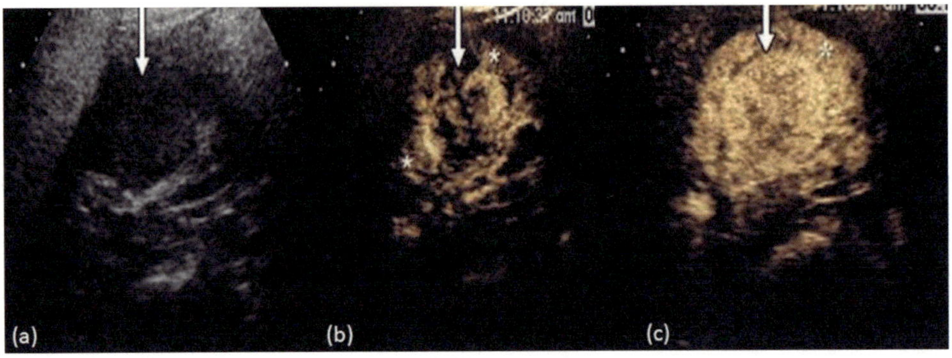

Figure 3.
(a) Gray scale imaging of renal mass showing hypo echoiec mass lesion at mid pole of right kidney (b) 16 seconds after contrast injection, heterogeneous enhancement (white arrow) which is higher than the adjacent renal parenchyma (*). (c) 19 seconds after contrast injection it shows uniform enhancement [13].

alone were not enough for the diagnosis and so, a combination of tumor heterogeneity with delayed contrast washout had specificity of 82% and positive predictive value of 85% for conventional ccRCC. At the same time hypo enhancing ccRCC are a challenge for diagnosis. Also, CEUS can reliably detect enhancing tumor thrombus within the renal vein.

2.1.2 Ultrasound molecular imaging

Molecular imaging is a highly innovative approach which involves targeting and real time, in vivo evaluation of physiological processes. As an extension of CEUS, molecular targeted micro bubbles are developed. Ideally response to ongoing systemic treatment is determined by changes in the volume of the tumor. Molecular imaging allows evaluation of changes in tumor physiology earlier than the tumor volume changes. This can help in earlier evaluation of tumor progression and response to treatment which aids in timely therapeutic decision making. Molecular imaging can characterize features like angiogenesis more potentially helping in treatment option choices. Many researchers have studied molecular imaging in mice models. They found the response to therapy detection was better for molecular imaging than with the volume measurements [14]. Molecular imaging has the potential for serial monitoring and assessment of disease response to systemic therapy, still it is in very early phases of development and much research is needed [1].

2.1.3 Elastography

Ultrasound elastography measures the tissue stiffness (which is present in diffuse parenchymal diseases) and the resultant tissue architectural changes. Strain elastography is a qualitative or semi qualitative evaluation of tissue elasticity using external compression and decompression cycles from the transducer. Shear wave elastography (SWE) is a quantitative assessment of tissue elasticity by measuring propagation speed of shear waves through the tissue. It does not require external compression and relies on a high amplitude push pulse known as acoustic radiation force impulse (ARFI). So it is less operator dependant. Strain elastography helps to aid in the discrimination of benign from malignant lesions, RCC from AML and RCC from transitional cell carcinoma (TCC). SWE also has potential value in differentiating various sub types of RCC, pseudo tumor and AML. However it cannot differentiate ccRCC from AML. Few studies have been done for its utility; however the value is limited in validation and application in renal mass characterization is limited at present. Omur et al. stated that mean strain index values are significantly higher in malignant lesions compared with benign solid renal lesions [15].

2.1.4 Micro Doppler techniques

Simple renal cysts show no evidence of internal vascularity due to clear contents as opposed to solid lesion. In such reasons, the pattern of vascularity may help in mass discrimination (malignancy versus pseudo tumor). Novel micro Doppler studies improve the detection of slow flow within the small diameter vessels which increases the ability to detect subtle vascularity within the lesion [16]. Conventional Doppler has threshold limits lower than such novel techniques. Advantages of such techniques are exclusion of the need of IV contrast medium. However the results have not been compared to that of CEUS. Further investigations and studies are needed for its implications.

2.2 CT scan

CT scan is the primary imaging technique for the diagnosis, staging, treatment planning and surveillance of RCC. Contrast enhanced CT scan is performed after intravenous injection of contrast medium. And then various phases are taken according to

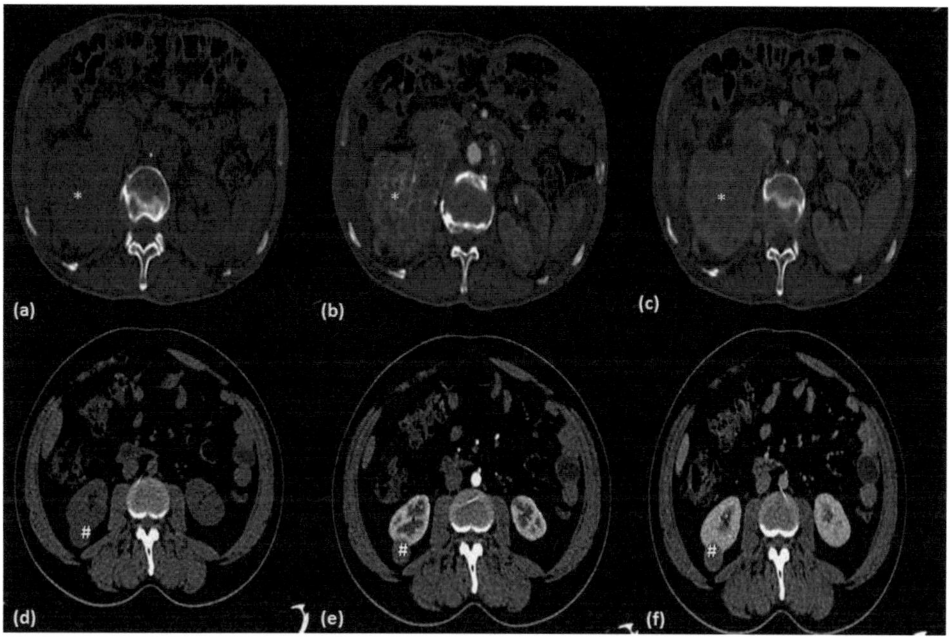

Figure 4.
(a-c) Axial CT imaging of right renal mass- clear cell carcinoma, showing enhancement pattern on various phases. (a) Non enhanced phase shows hypodense lesion in right kidney(*) (b) similar lesion enhances heterogeneously on arterial phase(*). Thrombus within renal vein and IVC is also noted (arrow). (c) Similar lesion shows contrast wash out on venous phase(*). (d-f) Axial CT imaging of right renal mass- papillary cell carcinoma, showing enhancement pattern on various phases. (d) Non enhanced phase shows hypodense lesion in right kidney(#). (e) Arterial phase shows minimal enhancement of the lesion(#). (f) Similar lesion shows increased enhancement on venous phase(#).

the time interval i.e. nephrographic phase, cortico medullary phase and delayed phase. Various sub types of RCC exhibit various patterns of enhancement in different phases of CECT scan; hence they can be differentiated accordingly. Clear cell RCC (most common subtype) is hyper vascular with heterogeneous texture and it enhances in nephrographic phase and the contrast washes out in corticomedullary phase; Papillary RCC is hypovascular so it enhances over the period of time with the phases (**Figure 4**); Oncocytoma shows almost similar pattern of enhancement however the central non enhancing scar is the characteristic feature of oncocytoma. Chromophobe RCC has intermediate vascularity and is usually well circumscribed. Another important finding in RCC to sought for is tumor thrombus involvement of renal vein and IVC. Venous extension of tumor in RCC is best seen in corticomedullary phase of CECT scan.

2.2.1 CT perfusion

CT perfusion allows visualization and quantification of blood perfusion in tissue. After iodine based contrast agent injection, low dose contrast enhanced CT scan images are achieved at multiple time intervals and the contrast passes through vessels and tissue. It allows quantitative analysis of blood flow, blood volume and mean transit time. The role of CT perfusion is well known for analysis of stroke; however, its role in abdominal solid tumor imaging like RCC is still in primary stages. Due to increased vascularity in RCC, it is easily visualized with CT perfusion (**Figure 5**). Most RCC treatments affect angiogenesis and targeted therapies have a greater effect on metastatic sites than on the primary tumor site. Targeted treatment reduces tumor vascularity, decreases proliferation and increases apoptosis and immune cell infiltration as

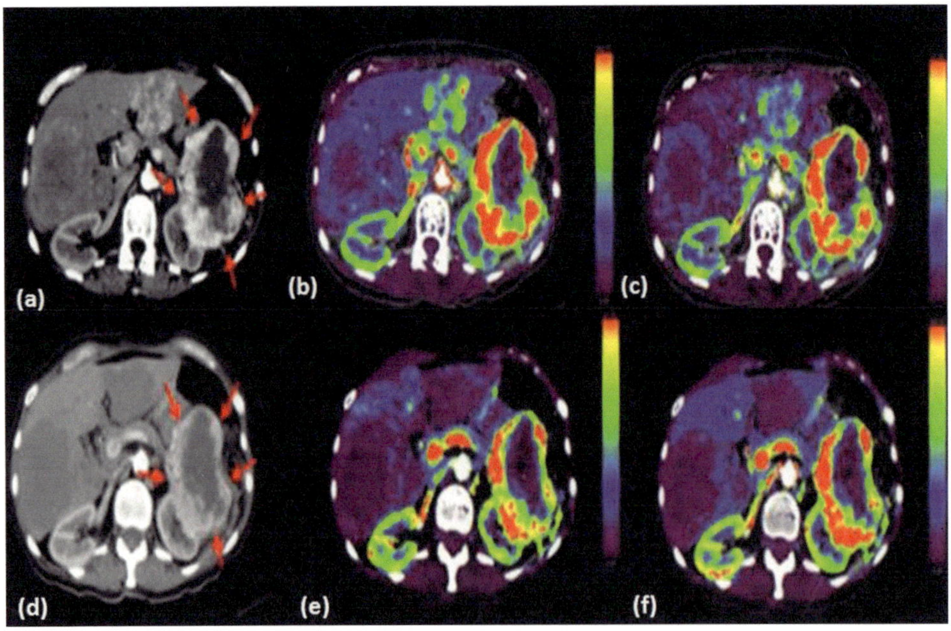

Figure 5.
(a-f) Axial images of contrast enhanced CT scan and perfusion of left renal mass. (a-c): Images of left renal mass before starting treatment (red arrows). Blood flow was 116 (±84.12) ml/100 ml/min and blood volume is 13.79 (± 7.79) ml/100 ml. (d-f) Similar patient at 8 days of starting treatment. The blood flow showed mild reduction to 100.13 (± 77.96) ml/100 ml/min and blood volume to 10.38 (±9.6) ml/100 ml [17].

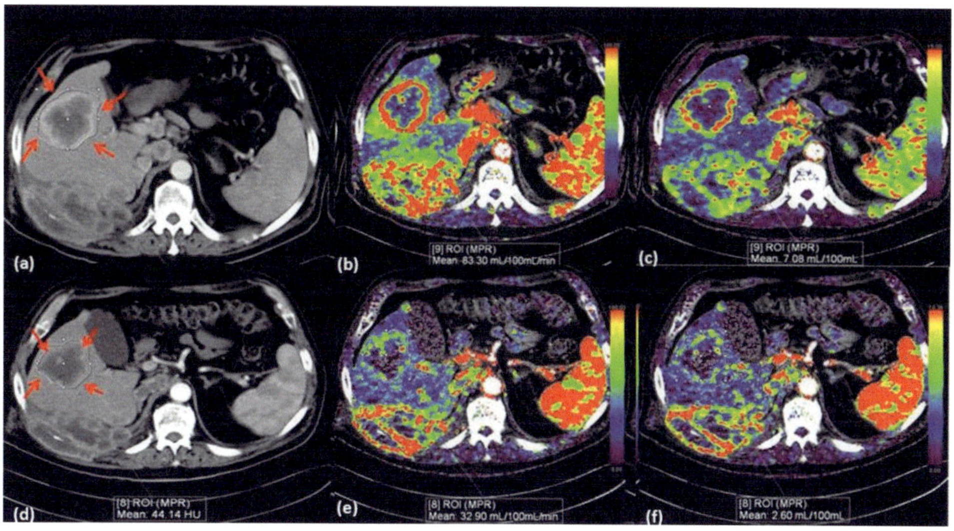

Figure 6.
(a-c): Axial imaging of contrast enhanced and perfusion CT scan of metastatic lesion in right lobe of liver before starting treatment (red arrows). Primary lesion is RCC. Blood flow was 83.3 (±70.48) ml/100 ml/min and blood volume is 7.08 (± 7.23) ml/100 ml. (d-f) Similar patient at 8 days of starting treatment. The blood flow reduced significantly to 32.90 (± 28.88) ml/100 ml/min and blood volume to 2.60 (±3.35) ml/100 ml [17].

early as 1 week after treatment initiation [17]. Treatment response determined through various bio markers can be assessed as early as 12 weeks after initiation of treatment. However, with the help of CT perfusion, this time can be reduced to as early as 1 to 2 weeks. Albeit, the majority of data have been published which have this latent time period of 5 to 10 weeks after initiation of treatment; more research is needed for the reduced time interval in such studies. In a highly metastatic tumor like advanced RCC; the main goal of systemic treatment is cessation of progression of tumor which can prevent the specific morbidity due to pain or hemorrhage. Alice et al. found larger reduction in blood volume in metastatic lesions than in primary lesions. They also stated that early perfusion changes in the metastatic lesions can determine the response of particular therapy (**Figure 6**) [17].

2.2.2 Dual energy CT scan (DECT)

DECT is newer type of CT scanner having two sets of x ray tubes with two different levels of energy which pass through the patient body. Interaction of these two energy x ray beam with the body tissue helps in material identification and quantification [18]. These two datasets at high and low energy helps in additional characterization of kidneys and urinary tract. DECT is also used to evaluate iodine and calcium concentrations and helps to differentiate pathological processes and evaluate internal structure of the lesion [19]. Minimal enhancing hypodense renal tumors can be differentiated from a cyst through iodine quantification which is a biomarker for tumor vascularity. Improved visibility of the lesion reduces the frequency of repeated follow up imaging. It also helps in assessment of tumor response in context of tumor vascularity and necrosis. DECT is capable of reducing the radiation dose by applying virtual non contrast images which eliminates the need for pre contrast imaging.

Papillary RCC has low vascularity and shows homogeneous and low enhancement compared to adjacent renal parenchyma on CT scan making it difficult to differentiate from more benign lesions like cyst. Iodine specific DECT allows color coded display of iodine inside the renal lesion facilitating differentiation of a non enhancing cyst from enhancing solid lesion easily. Sensitivity of iodine signal compensates for the poor enhancement of lesions such as papillary RCC and allows its accurate characterization [20]. DECT is also useful in evaluation of patients with polycystic kidney diseases (PCKD) with renal mass lesions. PCKD patients also have to undergo multiple follow up for extended period of time; in such cases DECT helps by offering reduced radiation dose. In post treatment (thermal ablation) renal lesions and in residual renal tumors; enhancement assessment (i.e a sign of viability) is difficult on conventional CT scan owing to changes due to ablation and perinephric bleeding. DECT with iodine mapping proves a valuable tool. Park et al. stated the diagnostic performance of DECT for predicting tumor progression in patients treated with Radio frequency ablation with sensitivity 100% and specificity 91.5% [21]. Normalizing iodine ratio with aorta reduces the variability due to different acquisition protocols. Also, iodine ratio was proposed to be an independent predictor for differentiating ccRCC from non ccRCC lesions (**Figure 7**) [22]. Given its better results in differentiating ccRCC from other subtypes, DECT may emerge as a novel technique for choosing patients for surveillance noninvasively.

2.2.3 CT texture analysis (CTTA)

Heterogeneity is the key feature of renal cell carcinoma. CT texture analysis is emerging tool to quantify tissue for heterogeneity in renal cell carcinoma which cannot be perceived through naked eye. It is a technology for automatically extracting quantitative parameters from the images of CT scan. It can extract plenty of features from each image and thus can provide more detailed information than conventional imaging [23]. It can differentiate fat poor AML from RCC [24]. It provides valuable information for grading, staging and predicting the prognosis of tumor. Conventional and contrast enhanced CT scan along with CTTA can non-invasively classify grades of RCC. However, detailed research is needed for better application of such technology.

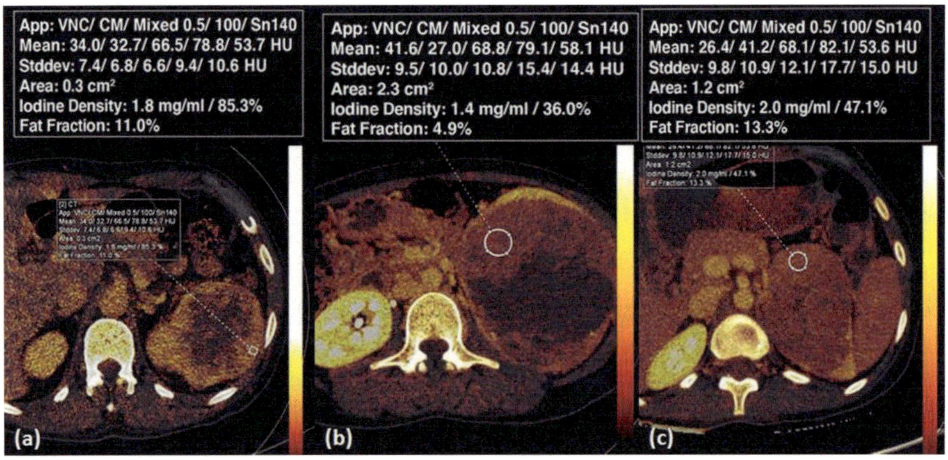

Figure 7.
Axial section of dual energy CT scan(DECT) image showing ccRCC, papillary RCC and Chromophobe RCC in left kidneys of three different patients. Iodine ratio (appears as iodine density in images) is 85.3% in ccRCC, 36% in papillary RCC and 47.1% in Chromophobe RCC. Circles denotes the region of interest in tumors [21].

CTTA avoids the subjective influence of image processing and reduces the errors. Conventional Imaging techniques assess the tumor in context of its size, shape and contrast enhancement which can only define the outline and cannot provide the grade of lesion. Subtle changes within the pixel intensity of the lesion occurring due to tumor heterogeneity in low and high grade RCC are picked up easily in CTTA. CTTA performs comprehensive evaluation of lesions and avoids sampling error.

2.2.4 Fast Fourier transform (FFT) analysis

FFT analysis helps to differentiate various solid non fat containing enhancing renal tumor on CT scan. It uses a quantitative parameter such as tumor attenuation which is extracted from multiphase CT scan. Such features also help in differentiating various renal tumor subtypes. Various parameters gained in FFT analysis are FFT magnitude (measuring diversity of measurements) and complexity index (CI). Entropy of FFP magnitude, entropy of FFP phase and complexity index is calculated for the final result and depending upon them inference is made. On applying FFT analysis to segmented tumor images, the magnitude spectrum of malignant tumors show increased intensity of frequencies whereas it is comparatively lower in benign lesions owing to the level of heterogeneity [25]. The FFT magnitude, FFT phase and CI entropy measurement is able to indentify grade I and IV tumors from the rest of them. However heterogeneity of ccRCC is higher papillary RCC in all grades.

CI index is helpful in differentiating ccRCC from oncocytoma in excretory phase where the CI is higher for ccRCC. Similarly lipid poor AML (lpAML) can be differentiated from oncocytoma with the help of entropy of FFG magnitude which is higher in lpAML than oncocytoma in excretory phase (**Figure 8**). lpAML shows rapid enhancement on corticomedullary phase with washout in excretory phase. Usually, the difference between lpAML and oncocytoma is most prominent in nephrographic and excretory phases. However, no significant differentiation between FFT metrics is noted between Chromophobe RCC and papillary RCC [25].

All the quantitative metrics can provide assessment of tumor heterogeneity to improve the diagnostic confidence. They are not useful alone, a combination of imaging features are a must. FFT metrics have a lower value in benign lesions and it can identify the differences between lpAML and oncocytoma from ccRCC. Additionally 3D analysis can also be possible which can help in regions to be targeted for biopsy.

2.3 MRI

Superior soft tissue contrast of MRI has a sensitivity and specificity in detecting and characterizing RCC comparable to contrast enhanced CT scan. It avoids the risk of ionizing radiation and helps to detect very small enhancing regions within complex cystic lesions. However it is less accessible, costly and takes a longer time for scanning. Along with CT thorax, MRI can be used for pre operative staging of RCC due to its yield of rich morphological and functional information. Renal MRI protocol includes non contrast enhanced T1 and T2 weighted sequences, chemical shift imaging for detection of fat and dynamic contrast enhanced 3D gradient echo sequences for tumoral contrast enhancement. Dynamic imaging can obtain corticomedullary, nephrographic and excretory phases. Coronal 3D fast gradient echo sequence with fat suppression after dynamic series facilitates imaging of renal venous anatomy and inferior vena cava (IVC) for evaluation of thrombus. Subtle enhancement within

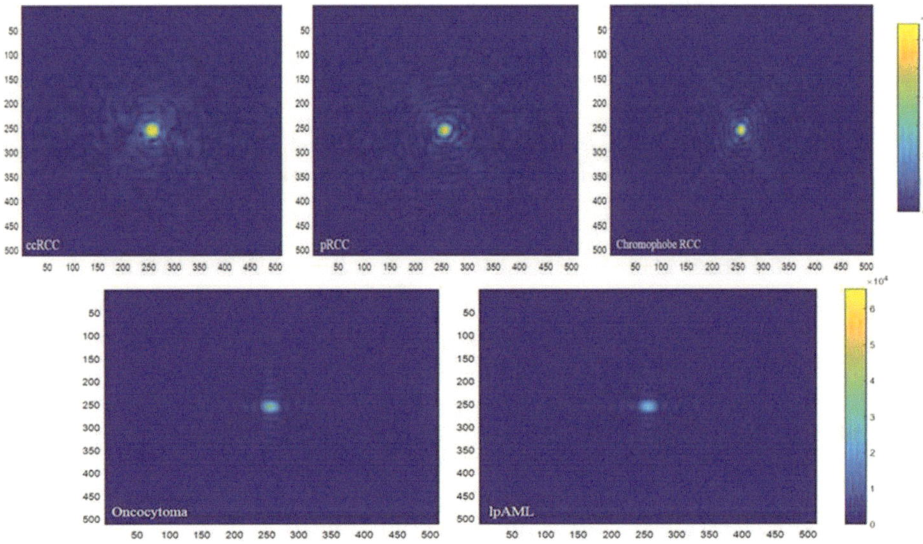

Figure 8.
Magnitude spectrum of malignant renal masses (upper row) and benign renal masses (lower row). High frequency in malignant tumors and lower in benign tumors is noted [25].

the mass lesion can be obtained with 3D gradient echo sequence due to its ability to subtract post and pre contrast images.

Various MRI features in different sequences can help to differentiate various RCC subtypes. Microscopic fat within the AML can be easily demonstrated by India ink artifacts surrounding the macroscopic fat in the mass on in and out of phase images [19]. T2 weighted sequence and post contrast sequence helps to characterize the complexity of cystic or necrotic RCC. ccRCC is seen as iso or hypo intense mass lesion as compared to its adjacent renal parenchyma on pre contrast T1 weighted sequences and appears as heterogeneously hyperintense on T2 weighted sequences. ccRCC show intense heterogeneous enhancement on cortico medullary phase MRI unlike other RCC subtypes. ccRCC also appears as hypointense on T2 weighted sequences on excretory phases with rapid wash out of contrast medium. Papillary RCC is homogeneously low signal intensity on T2 weighted sequences due to intra tumoral hemosiderin and shows low enhancement on contrast enhanced dynamic sequences. ccRCC showed more intensity changes than papillary RCC on corticomedullary and nephrographic phase images (**Figure 9**). However, it has been stated that signal intensity changes on corticomedullary phases are most reliable parameter for differentiating ccRCC and papillary RCC [27]. Various quantitative techniques e.g. arterial spin labeling (ASL), diffusion weighted imaging (DWI) and intra voxel incoherent motion (IVIM) have the ability to assess vascularity within the tumor and can be useful for differentiating between various RCC subgroups and in post treatment surveillance.

2.3.1 MR perfusion

MR perfusion is a technique measuring vascularity (perfusion) of the tissue after the injection of contrast agent. Where multi parametric MRI can assess enhancement of the tissue, MR perfusion gives quantitative parameters. Signal intensity curves are generated and placed against time and post processing is done to achieve perfusion

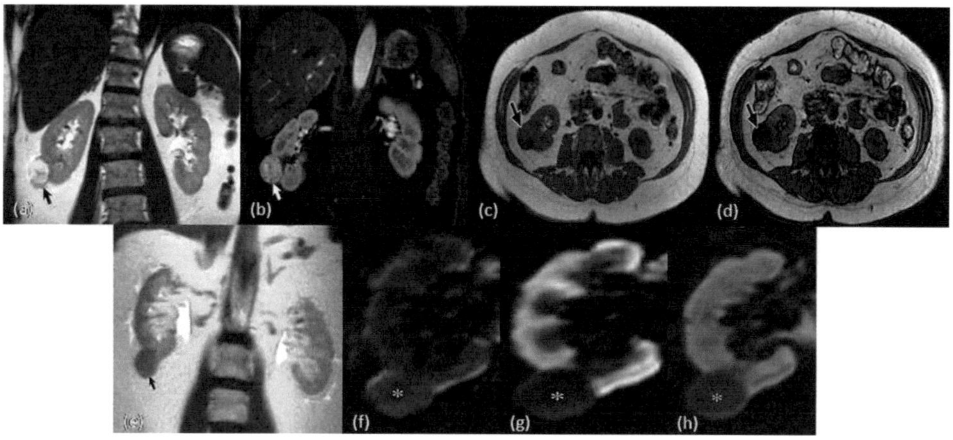

Figure 9.
(a-d) MRI images showing ccRCC. (a) Coronal non fat saturated T2 weighted single shot fast spin echo images showing high signal intensity renal mass arising from right kidney lower pole (black arrow). (b) Coronal contrast enhanced corticomedullary fat saturated T1 weighted gradient recalled echo MR image showing high contrast enhancement within the lesion (white arrow). (c) Axial in phase and (d) axial out of phase non fat saturated T1 weighted gradient recalled echo MR images. Signal dropout is seen on image (d) in comparison to image (c) denoting presence of intra voxel fat. (e-h) MRI images showing papillary RCC. (e) Coronal non fat saturated T2 weighted single shot fast spin echo MR image showing low signal intensity lesion at lower pole of right kidney (black arrow). Coronal T1 weighted fat saturated spoiled gradient recalled echo MR images in pre contrast (f), corticomedullary phase(g) and nephrographic phase (h) of similar lesion (*). Low contrast enhancement is seen in corticomedullary (g) and nephrographic phases (h) [26].

parameters. Tissue perfusion can also be achieved without contrast agent in arterial spin labeling technique (ASL). In ASL, red blood cells (RBCs) are used as endogenous contrast agent that is labeled non invasively with MR gradient and radio frequency and then perfusion within the tissue is calculated with the help of inflow of labeled RBCs. The use of endogenous contrast eliminates the erroneous calculation due to vascular permeability and it can also be done in patients with contraindications to MR contrast agents. However it has low sensitivity in hypo vascular tumors. Tumor grading in RCC can also be done with MR perfusion. Higher grade RCC shows higher perfusion values. In anti cholinergic drug therapy administered for metastatic RCC; changes in vascularity are achieved before the changes in the size of tumor and thus early response assessment can be done [28].

2.3.2 Diffusion weighted MRI

Diffusion weighted (DWI) is a functional imaging which uses random motion of water particles. (Brownian motion). The extent of vascularity within the tissue as well as presence of an intact cell membrane is the features which determine the impedance of diffusion of water molecule. That is quantified by apparent diffusion coefficient (ADC) maps. If the diffusion of water molecule is restricted, ADC value is less e.g. in tumor cells with dysfunctional cell membranes. DWI can detect cellular changes in the tissue before traditional imaging. Zhang H et al. reported the significant difference of ADC with pooled weighted sensitivity 88% and specificity of 72% in a study assessing DWI's ability to differentiate benign from malignant masses [29]. ADC values for ccRCC and oncocytoma are higher compared to papillary RCC due to their high vascularity. However no significant ADC value difference is seen between ccRCC and oncocytoma (**Figure 10**). Conventional ADC value derived from single slice ROI

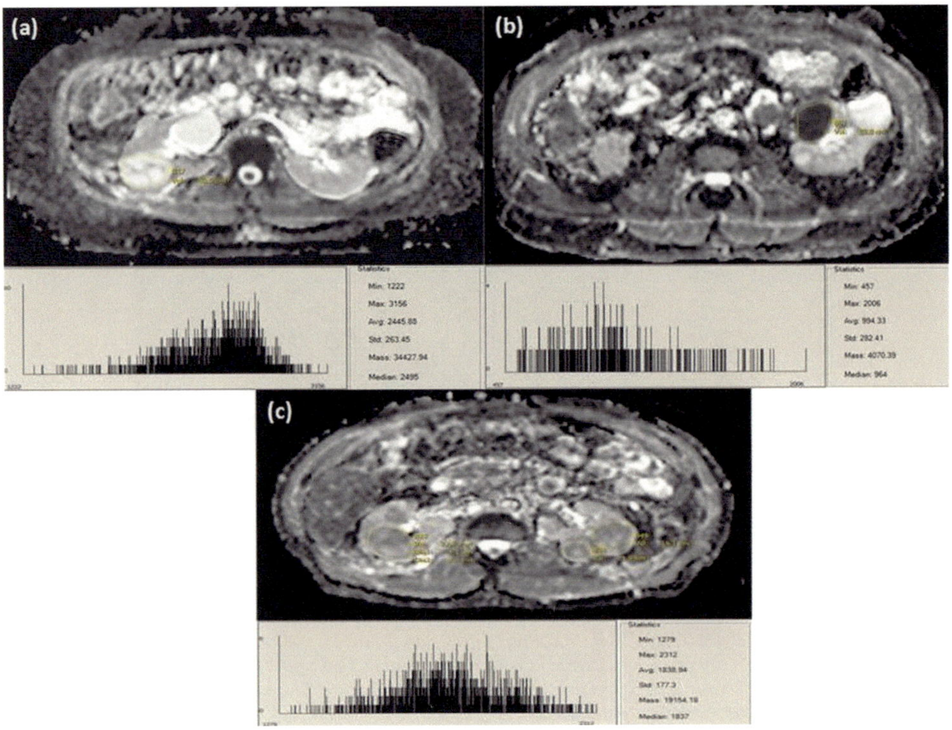

Figure 10.
ADC map and histogram of (a) ccRCC (b) papillary RCC and (c) oncocytoma lesions [30].

is less accurate than near technique where whole lesion analysis is done. Whole lesion analysis helps to evaluate tumor structure and histology more accurately. Distribution of ADC values on histogram helps the radiologist to identify the heterogeneous features of the lesion which are more common to ccRCC or oncocytoma as compared to papillary RCC [30]. Mean ADC values derived from small region of interest (ROI) within the tumor have been studied for differentiation of renal tumors. IVIM and diffusion kurtosis are newer quantitative parameters helping in differentiating renal benign from malignant masses and also help in grading of RCC. IVIM is bi exponential parameter including true as well as pseudo diffusion. It calculates various parameters like diffusivity (D), pseudo diffusion coefficient (D*) and perfusion index (F). A significant variation is noted in diffusion kurtosis parameters between various RCC subtypes and grades [28].

2.3.3 Bold

BOLD is non invasive quick MRI sequence evaluating deoxyhemoglobin level in the kidney. The oxygen tension in kidneys varies with the blood flow as well as with the need for the filtration. Cortex of the kidney is perfused well and is high in oxygen levels whereas medullary region is relatively less perfused and shows low oxygen tension. As a result there is higher production of deoxyhemoglobin. Deoxyhemoglobin has a para magnetic effects and causes rapid photon dephasing. Decreased T2 relaxation time is achieved due to higher amount of deoxyhemoglobin [28]. BOLD MRI has established role in brain imaging. Various renal lesions would show altered perfusion in the kidney so BOLD MRI can be a helping tool for differentiating benign from malignant renal lesions. However, still renal application of BOLD MRI has to undergo a lot of research.

2.3.4 Proton spectroscopy

Proton spectroscopy (H1MRS) is a newer technology studying various chemical metabolic agents in determining various pathologies. It studies chemical compositions and metabolic processes *in vivo*. The changes in Larmor frequency within the magnetic field is due to differing chemical composition, which is called "chemical shift". As of now the established role of Proton spectroscopy is in imaging of central nervous system, breast and prostatic regions [28]. However Kim et al. studied five patients with biopsy proven RCC and found the difference of lipid and choline as per the tumor grade (**Figure 11**) [31]. However, MR spectroscopy has various limitations also i.e. complexity of acquisition, processing and data interpretation. It has low sensitivity and poor spatial resolution. Hence it can only be used as complementary technique for basic MRI.

2.4 Single photon emission computed tomography (SPECT)

SPECT is used in various clinical settings including living kidney donation, surveillance of renal function during chemotherapy or in patients for endo radiotherapy. An agent ^{99m}Tc-Sestamibi is an established tracer used for cardiac applications which is highly specific for mitochondria. Due to increased amount of mitochondria in the renal oncocytoma lesions, role of ^{99m}Tc-Sestamibi can be rationalized for differentiating various renal masses. ^{99m}Tc-Sestamibi SPECT/CT has sensitivity and specificity

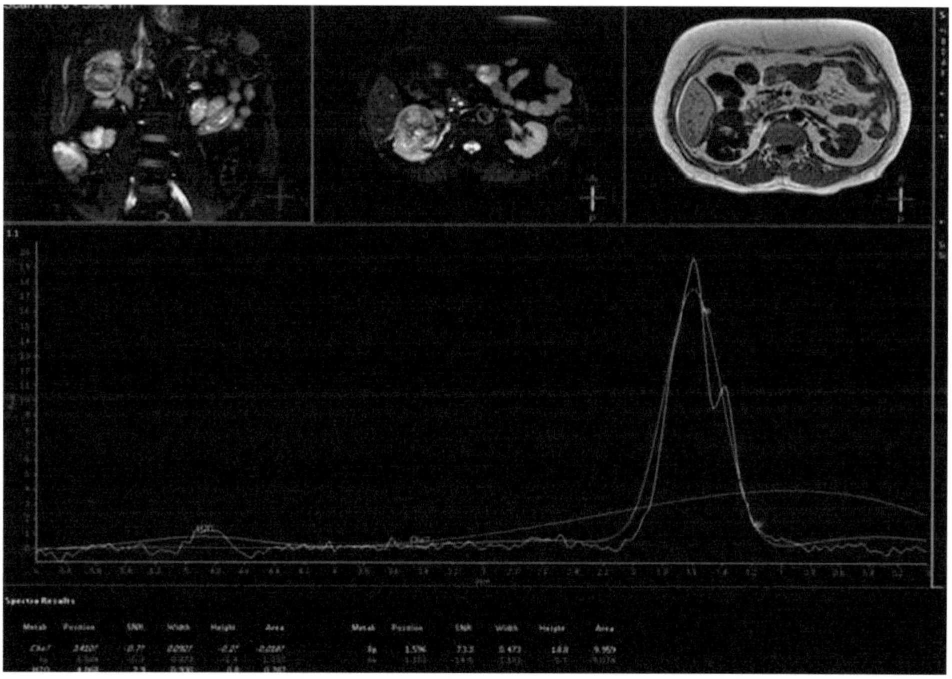

Figure 11.
MR spectroscopy of low grade RCC showing increased lipid lactate peak [28].

of more than 87% to differentiate between renal oncocytoma and oncocytoma/ Chromophobe masses versus RCC. However due to multiple advantages of PET scan, it has overruled the use of SPECT in renal lesions [32].

2.5 Positron emission tomography (PET) scan

Improved absolute quantification, improved spatiotemporal resolution and simultaneous acquisition for attenuation correction and anatomic co-registration are major advantages of PET scan over SPECT [32]. PET scan using fluoro deoxyglucose (FDG) is a functional imaging detecting various malignancies through observation of glucose uptake and rate of glycolysis in neoplastic tissue. It is useful in restaging of RCC and to detect metastatic lesions. However, it is less satisfactory in detection of primary diseases. The major excretion route for FDG is kidneys and thus an unfavorable back ground activity is seen which hinders the results making it less preferable for detection of primary renal lesions. Papillary RCC shows high avidity for FDG. ccRCC variant shows limited FDG uptake and so, non FDG molecular agents need to be evaluated for their use in other subtypes of RCC [19]. Higher FDG intake in to tumor thrombus compared to bland thrombus indicates another use of FDG in patients with RCC. Wang HY et al. reported overall sensitivity and specificity of FDG PET as 79% and 90% in identification of extrarenal lesions respectively [33]. Alongi et al. stated the sensitivity of FDG imaging to be 74% and specificity 80% and also stated that FDG positive cases resulted in significantly lower (69%) five year survival rates compared to FDG negative cases (19%) [34]. FDG PET can detect larger lesions compared to smaller ones and also can detect higher grade masses more easily than low grade masses. Various other PET scan agents are also identified and some of them are superior to FDG in various aspects.

^{18}F labeled anti-1-amino-3-[^{18}F]-flurocyclobutane-1-carboxylic acid (anti-^{18}F-FACBC) is useful in differentiating papillary RCC from ccRCC. PSMA targeting radio tracer agent ^{18}F-DCFPyL provides highly specific use in ccRCC. ^{68}Ga labeled PSMA PET shows higher sensitivity for detection of metastasis in RCC. ^{18}F-PSMA-1007 also has been applied to test its capability for surveillance in metastatic RCC.

^{18}F-Fluoromisonidazole (FMISO) PET is used for evaluation of tumors which are hypoxic and show poor response to targeted therapy. ^{18}F-Fluorothymidine (FLT) PET can differentiate inflammation from tumors more accurately than ^{18}F-FDG. ^{11}C acetate PET can be used in primary renal lesions. ^{18}F-fluoroethylcholine PET is used for evaluation of metastatic RCC. ^{68} Ga-PSMA PET is very effectively being used in patients with Carcinoma Prostate, it is most widely investigated tracer for RCC also [35]. However, the role of PET scan in detection of primary renal lesions is not significant. Hence, advanced modalities like PET CT and PET MRI are being studied for their role in RCC.

2.5.1 PET/CT scan

Physiological excretion of ^{18}FDG via the kidneys makes it difficult to evaluate renal lesions with the background of high FDG activity. However FDG PET can reveal various differences in metabolic activity based on histological subtypes of RCC. To acquire advantages of both these imaging technologies, hybrid advance imaging combining PET scan with CT scan has been evolved. The physiological advantages of PET scan are combined with anatomical images of CT scan and the superimposed image can correlate the high activity regions with the anatomical site making diagnosis

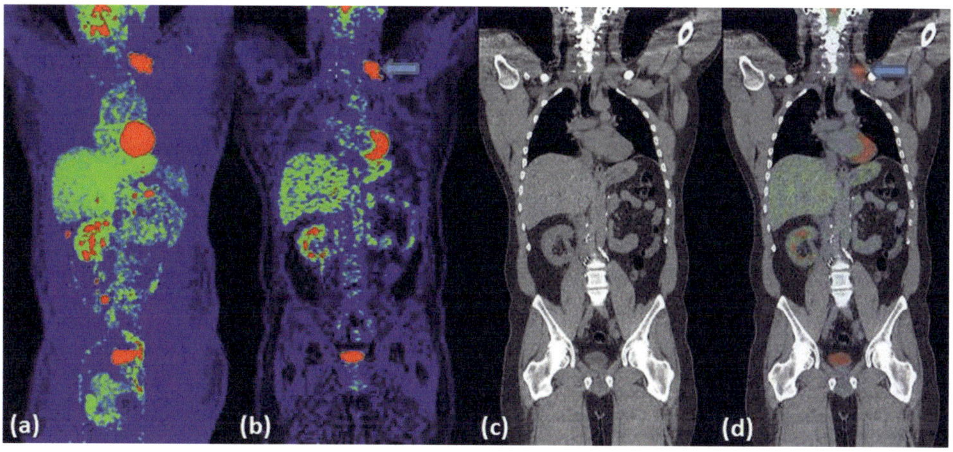

Figure 12.
(a) FDG PET MIP image of patient with RCC (b) coronal PET image (c) coronal CT scan image and (d) PET/CT scan fusion image of similar patient. Left supra clavicular regional metastatic lymph nodes are clearly visualized in PET/CT scan (blue arrow) which was not seen on CT scan (c) [19].

more accurate. Hybrid PET CT scanners eliminate the disadvantage of two separate scanners for PET and CT scans and combine both the modalities in single scanner (**Figure 12**). That results in improved anatomical demarcation along with improved diagnosis of post operative scar tissue, surgical clips and relations with surrounding organs [35]. Many authors have proposed that a predictor called standardized uptake value (SUV) in PET scan is a significant predictor for Fuhrman's grading of RCC [35]. A SUV value cutoff of 3.0 can differentiate between low and high grade ccRCC with sensitivity 89% and specificity 87%. ccRCC shows higher SUV than chromophobe RCC. However, Chromophobe RCC is very difficult to differentiate from oncocytoma lesions even with hybrid PET CT scan.

Quantitative measurement like SUV in FDG PET/CT can play a role in prediction of the tumor progression by objective estimation of biological behavior of tumor. Namura et al. evaluated the impact of SUVmax on survival in advanced RCC patients. They concluded high SUVmax to correlate with poor prognosis [36]. High grade tumor show intense tracer uptake and a higher SUV. SUVmax exceeding 10 was associated with the highest rate of mortality [37]. As high grade primary RCC with high SUVmax has high chances of occult metastasis. Thus FDG PET/CT helps to predict the extrarenal disease. Sensitivity and specificity of FDG PET was ranging from 63–75% and 90–100% respectively when compared to CECT scan in detection of extra renal pelvis [35]. PET/CT scan is less accurate to assess metastatic lesions measuring less than 5 mm in lungs and liver. However, for detection of metastatic lesions in bone and adrenal glands, FDG PET/CT scan is very sensitive. FDG PET/CT scan showed high predictive value in surveillance of targeted therapy.

2.5.2 Pet/MRI

PET/MRI combines the advantages of anatomical localization and attenuation correction map for quantification of PET images through concurrent acquisition. It uses the same reference frame which helps to overlay the *in vivo* independent structural, functional and metabolic features of the tumor. Most widely used method for assessment of therapy response is Response Evaluation Criteria in Solid Tumors

(RECIST v1.1). It is dependent on one dimension measurements on imaging for tumor diameter and RECIST v1.1 may not be able to detect early responses on imaging. Here, advanced technologies like PET/MRI can play a useful role. Various obstacles have been experienced in diagnosis made with PET/MRI like, different imaging sequences have to be transformed in to voxel wise correspondence for spatial heterogeneity, to eliminate or correct acquisition artifacts due to movement and image parameter drift and visual assessment of data. This issue can be overcome with computer extracted parameter from radiological images which is known as radiomics [38]. Radiomics captures the image texture through quantification of changes in signal intensity within the tumor which can be due to early treatment response. These features can be missed visually.

3. Summary

Multi modality imaging is advised for pre treatment diagnosis, discrimination of various subtypes and post treatment surveillance of RCC. Conventional imaging techniques at times falls short for proper diagnostic information. Advanced hybrid techniques are being evaluated a lot these days and they will provide a lot more information in future. Detailed study is being executed in various modalities which will be helpful for better characterization of renal cell carcinoma and its subtypes.

Author details

Vaidehi Alpesh Patel
Department of Radio-Diagnosis, G. R. Doshi and K.M. Mehta Institute of Kidney Diseases and Research Centre (IKDRC), Dr. H. L. Trivedi Institute of Transplantation Sciences (ITS), Gujarat University of Transplantation Sciences, Civil Hospital Campus, Asarwa, Ahmedabad, Gujarat, India

*Address all correspondence to: drvaidehipandya@gmail.com

References

[1] Roussel E, Campi R, Amparore D, Bertolo R, Carbonara U, Erdem S, et al. Expanding the role of ultrasound for the characterization of renal masses. Journal of Clinical Medicine. 2022;**11**:1112

[2] van Oostenbrugge TJ, Spenkelink IM, Bokacheva L, Rusinek H, van Amerongen MJ, Langenhuijsen JF, et al. Kidney tumor diffusion-weighted magnetic resonance imaging derived ADC histogram parameters combined with patient characteristics and tumor volume to discriminate oncocytoma from renal cell carcinoma. European Journal of Radiology. 2021;**145**:110013

[3] Feng Z, Shen Q, Li Y, Zhengyu H. CT texture analysis: A potential tool for predicting the Fuhrman grade of clear-cell renal carcinoma. Cancer Imaging. 2019;**19**(a):6

[4] Dwivedi DK, Xi Y, Kapur P, Madhuranthakam AJ, Lewis M, Udayakumar D, et al. MR imaging Radiomics analyses for prediction of high grade histology and necrosis in clear cell renal cell carcinoma: Preliminary experience. Clinical Genitourinary Cancer. 2021;**19**(1):12-21

[5] Razik A, Goyal A, Sharma R, Kandasamy D, Seth A, Das P, et al. MR texture analysis in differentiating renal cell carcinoma from lipid-poor angiomyolipoma and oncocytoma. The British Journal of Radiology. 2020;**93**(1114):20200569

[6] Zhu A h, Hou X y, Tian S, Zhang W f. Diagnostic value of 18F-FDG PET/CT versus contrast enhanced MRI for venous tumour thrombus and venous bland thrombus in renal cell carcinoma. Scientific Reports. 2022;**12**(1):587

[7] Morshid A, Duran ES, Choi WJ, et al. A concise review of the multimodality imaging features of renal cell carcinoma. Cureus. 2021;**13**(2):e13231

[8] Pysz MA, Willmann JK. Targeted contrast-enhanced ultrasound: An emerging technology in abdominal and pelvic imaging. Gastroenterology. 2011;**140**(3):785-790

[9] Gulati M, King KG, Gill IS, et al. Contrast-enhanced ultrasound (CEUS) of cystic and solid renal lesions: A review. Abdominal Imaging. 2015;**40**:1982-1996

[10] Furrer MA, Spycher SCJ, Büttiker SM, Gross T, Bosshard P, Thalmann GN, et al. Comparison of the diagnostic performance of contrast-enhanced ultrasound with that of contrast-enhanced computed tomography and contrast-enhanced magnetic resonance imaging in the evaluation of renal masses: A systematic review and meta-analysis. Eur. Urol. Oncol. 2020;**3**:464-473

[11] Zhou L, Tang L, Yang T, Chen W. Comparison of contrast-enhanced ultrasound with MRI in the diagnosis of complex cystic renal masses: A meta-analysis. Acta Radiologica. 2018;**59**:1254-1263

[12] Zhang F, Li R, Li G, Jin L, Shi Q, Du L. Value of contrast-enhanced ultrasound in the diagnosis of renal cancer and in comparison with contrast-enhanced computed tomography: A meta-analysis. Journal of Ultrasound in Medicine. 2019;**38**:903-914

[13] Gerst S, Hann LE, Li D, Gonen M, Tickoo S, Sohn MJ, et al. Evaluation of renal masses with contrast-enhanced ultrasound: Initial experience. AJR. 2011;**197**:897-906

[14] Rojas JD, Lin F, Chiang Y-C, Chytil A, Chong DC, Bautch VL, et al. Ultrasound molecular imaging of VEGFR-2 in clear-cell renal cell carcinoma tracks disease response to antiangiogenic and notch-inhibition therapy. Theranostics. 2018;**8**:141-155

[15] Onur MR, Poyraz AK, Bozgeyik Z, Onur AR, Orhan I. Utility of semiquantitative strain elastography for differentiation between benign and malignant solid renal masses. Journal of Ultrasound in Medicine. 2015;**34**:639-647

[16] Leong JY, Wessner CE, Kramer MR, Forsberg F, Halpern EJ, Lyshchik A, et al. Superb microvascular imaging improves detection of vascularity in indeterminate renal masses. J. Ultrasound. Med. Off. J. Am. Inst. Ultrasound. Med. 2020;**39**:1947-1955

[17] Fan AC, Sundaram V, Kino A, Schmiedeskamp H, Metzner TJ, Kamaya A. Early changes in CT perfusion parameters: Primary renal carcinoma versus metastases after treatment with targeted therapy. Cancers. 2019;**11**:608

[18] De Cecco CN, Darnell A, Rengo M, Muscogiuri G, Bellini D, Ayuso C, et al. Dual-energy CT: Oncologic applications. AJR American journal of roentgenology. 2012;**199**:S98-s105

[19] Bagheri MH, Ahlman MA, Lindenberg L, Turkbey B, Jeffrey Lind A, Civelek C. Advances in medical imaging for the diagnosis and management of common genitourinary cancers. Urologic Oncology. 2017;**35**(7):473-491

[20] Alanee S, Dynda DI, Hemmer P, Schwartz B. Low enhancing papillary renal cell carcinoma diagnosed by using dual energy computerized tomography: A case report and review of literature. Alanee et al. BMC Urology. 2014;**14**:102

[21] Park J, Chandarana H, Macari M, Megibow AJ. Dual-energy computed tomography applications in uroradiology. Current Urology Reports. 2012;**13**(1):55-62

[22] Manoharan D, Netaji A, Diwan K, Sharma S. Normalized dual-energy iodine ratio best differentiates renal cell carcinoma subtypes among quantitative imaging biomarkers from perfusion CT and dual-energy CT. AJR. 2020;**215**:1389-1397

[23] Wei Y, Liang G, Zeng L, Yang Y, Yinghua W. Accuracy of CT texture analysis for differentiating low-grade and high-grade renal cell carcinoma: Systematic review and meta-analysis. BMJ Open. 2021;**11**:e051470

[24] Zhang G-M-Y, Shi B, Xue H-D, Ganeshan B, Sun H, Jin Z-Y. Can quantitative CT texture analysis be used to differentiate subtypes of renal cell carcinoma? Clinical Radiology. 2019;**74**(4):287-294

[25] Varghese BA, Chen F, Hwang DH, Cen SY, Gill IS, Duddalwar VA. Differentiating solid, non-macroscopic fat containing, enhancing renal masses using fast Fourier transform analysis of multiphase CT. The British Journal of Radiology. 2018;**91**:20170789

[26] Kay FU, Canvasser NE, Xi Y, Pinho DF, Costa DN, de Leon AD, et al. Diagnostic performance and inter reader agreement of a standardized MR imaging approach in the prediction of small renal mass histology. Radiology. 2018;**287**(2):543-553

[27] Hallscheidt PJ, Bock M, Riedasch G, et al. Diagnostic accuracy of staging renal cell carcinomas using multidetector-row computed tomography and magnetic resonance imaging: A prospective study with histopathologic correlation. Journal

of Computer Assisted Tomography. 2004;**28**:333-339

[28] Aggarwal A, Das CJ, Sharma S. Recent advances in imaging techniques of renal masses. World Journal of Radiology. 2022;**14**(6):137-150

[29] Zhang H, Gan Q, Wu Y, Liu R, Liu X, Huang Z, et al. Diagnostic performance of diffusion-weighted magnetic resonance imaging in differentiating human renal lesions (benignity or malignancy): A meta-analysis. Abdom Radiol (NY). 2016;**41**:1997-2010

[30] Paschall AK, Mojdeh Mirmomen S, Symons R, Pourmorteza A, Gautam R, Sahai A, et al. Differentiating papillary type I RCC from clear cell RCC and oncocytoma: Application of whole-lesion volumetric ADC measurement. Abdom Radiol (NY). 2018;**43**(9):2424-2430

[31] Kim DY, Kim KB, Kim OD, Kim JK. Localized in vivo proton spectroscopy of renal cell carcinoma in human kidney. Journal of Korean Medical Science. 1998;**13**:49-53

[32] Rudolf AW, Pomper MG, Buck AK, Rowe SP, Higuchi T. SPECT and PET radiotracers in renal imaging. Seminars in Nuclear Medicine. 2022;**52**:406-418

[33] Wang HY, Ding HJ, Chen JH, Chao CH, Lu YY, Lin WY, et al. Meta-analysis of the diagnostic performance of [18F]FDG-PET and PET/CT in renal cell carcinoma. Cancer Imaging. 2012;**12**:464-474

[34] Alongi P, Picchio M, Zattoni F, Spallino M, Gianolli L, Saladini G, et al. Recurrent renal cell carcinoma: Clinical and prognostic value of FDG PET/CT. European Journal of Nuclear Medicine and Molecular Imaging. 2016;**43**:464-473

[35] Jena R, Narain TA, Singh UP, Srivastava A. Role of positron emission tomography/computed tomography in the evaluation of renal cell carcinoma. Indian J Urol. 2021;**37**(2):125-132

[36] Namura K, Minamimoto R, Yao M, Makiyama K, Murakami T, Sano F, et al. Impact of maximum standardized uptake value (SUVmax) evaluated by 18-Fluoro-2-deoxy-D-glucose positron emission tomography/computed tomography (18F-FDG-PET/CT) on survival for patients with advanced renal cell carcinoma: A preliminary report. BMC Cancer. 2010;**10**:667

[37] Ferda J, Ferdova E, Hora M, Hes O, Finek J, Topolcan O, et al. 18F-FDG-PET/CT in potentially advanced renal cell carcinoma: A role in treatment decisions and prognosis estimation. Anticancer Research. 2013;**33**:2665-2672

[38] Antunes J, Viswanath S, Rusu M, Valls L, Hoimes C, Avril N, et al. Radiomics analysis on FLT-PET/MRI for characterization of early treatment response in renal cell carcinoma: A proof-of- concept study. Translational Oncology. 2016;**9**(2):155-162